# Cupid's Challenge

# Cupid's Challenge

■ ■ ■

*Cupid's Challenge: Embracing, Restoring Love, Affection, Intimacy and Respect Through the Challenges of Chronic Pain*

*Liza H. Leal, M.D.*

Foreword by Duncan G. Foulds, D.D.S.

Waterside Productions

Printed in the United States of America

First Printing, 2021

ISBN-13: 978-1-951805-62-3 print edition
ISBN-13: 978-1-951805-63-0 ebook edition

Waterside Productions
2055 Oxford Ave
Cardiff, CA 92007
www.waterside.com

# Dedication

*To Duncan, my husband and best friend.*

*Words cannot express the blessing that you are. Every day is a gift with you in my life. I cherish your love, wisdom, kindness and your companionship. You are the love of my life.*

*To Denali, our fur child*
*You are the example of unconditional love!*

# Acknowledgements

Over the years, I have learned much from my family, patients and colleagues, and a wish to share their accumulated words of wisdom in this work. It is my hope to that you will be inspired as I have been inspired, by the people who have been vulnerable and contributed the most unbridled intimate conversations of their life, making this book possible and making it possible to share with others.

Thank you to my biggest fan, mentor, business partner, best friend and lover my husband, Duncan G. Foulds, D.D.S. for his inspiration and enormous wisdom that he shares openly.

I also wish to express my heart felt gratitude to Harvey McCloud, for his brilliant guidance and collaboration. The acuity, diligence and humor with which he approached the project have been pivotal at every step.

My sincere appreciation to the people at Waterside Production, who have worked assiduously on behalf of this book. Bill Gladstone, thank you for your direction and belief in this project.

Words cannot express the gratitude to the entire Meridian Health Institute team and patient family, your encouragement, feedback and assistance are a blessing. You are all my family.

Finally, to my family The Leal-Foulds Tribe – thank you for all of your love and support. Li-Li Doc and Papa Doc love you!

# Table of Contents

# Foreword

Duncan G. Foulds, D.D.S.

Tens of millions of Americans struggle every day with chronic pain. The culprits are many: arthritis, migraines, cancer, back pain, and worn joints, just to name a few. Though each individual's struggle with pain is intensely personal, it also impacts the people who are close to them, including their closest relationships and particularly their partner. Frequently, when chronic pain invades a marriage or partnership, one of the first things to change is the couple's intimate relationship, both physically and emotionally, as they confront the pain that one or both experience in their encounters. For many couples, the physical relationship that has been a mainstay of their love and affection is suddenly challenged. What always brought them pleasure now causes them pain. In addition, emotional pain often results in the form of embarrassment, anxiety, distance, confusing expectations, unintentional mis-messaging, anger, and hurt feelings.

Now, with the publication of *Cupid's Challenge*, Dr. Liza Leal takes on the important task of teaching people how to achieve intimate pleasure and fulfillment in the face of chronic pain. By doing so, she shines a bright and revealing light on an issue too often hidden deep in the shadows. In *Cupid's Challenge*, Liza writes about genuine people, real pain, and practical methods to deal with that pain and its results—methods that can help them recapture the joy, intimacy, and love that she believes every couple deserves.

As a cosmetic and reconstructive dentist for more than thirty years, I have developed a broad understanding of how to address and successfully manage pain. What most people don't realize is that a significant amount of chronic dental pain relief can be achieved by simply visiting a dentist who specializes in restorative and reconstructive treatment. I have seen my patients' marriages and relationships almost come to an end because one person is miserable, frustrated, and at their wit's end trying to deal with or manage pain resulting from head and neck aches, TMJ, migraines, all the way down to back and joint pain. TMJ is a great example of how pain can directly affect a relationship. When a person has severe TMJ, it becomes tiring and difficult to talk on the phone, or even kiss, much less enjoy the passionate kissing that is the "foreplay" for further intimacy. It was my journey in pain management that led me to cross paths with Liza.

She was inspired to write *Cupid's Challenge* based on her own life experiences. In her third year of medical school, she saw opportunity everywhere she looked, until she realized she was not feeling well herself. Like most doctors, she dismissed it and attributed it to working and studying too hard. Then, within months, she found herself in a wheelchair, diagnosed with a particularly destructive form of rheumatoid arthritis that was expected to keep her in constant pain and heavily medicated for the rest of her life. Subsequently, Liza then had two episodes where she was hospitalized and not expected to survive. But even though she did, she was told she would never be able to walk again. Despite this prognosis, she did not let her condition defeat her. Instead, she persevered spending the rest of her medical school training and residency in a wheelchair, often in severe pain, depressed, sedentary, and with her weight escalating by seventy pounds.

This is when we crossed paths and I became her newfound mentor, coaching her through her last years of residency and challenging her mindset and her approach to pain. When people are in pain, they often need an objective voice to come alongside of them, to hold them accountable, and speak encouragement into their lives. It took courage, faith, and sometimes hard-headed determination for Liza to stop feeling like a victim and transform her outlook into one of knowing and believing that she would walk again. She then took her recovery up one more notch to seeing herself not just as a chronic pain survivor but as a THRIVER.

If you were to meet Liza today, you would never believe that this attractive woman, bursting with energy, was the same person condemned many years ago by conventional medicine to a short life in either agony or a drug-induced haze. Today, other than having a slight limp when she climbs stairs, she is healthy and happy, embracing the world with great enthusiasm, hope, and determination.

Self-reliance and self-motivation are extremely important in managing pain, yet it often takes help to move forward and overcome the agony. And this is why Liza and I share a practice today where we are able to change peoples' lives, giving them hope and help to not just survive, but thrive every day in their activities and relationships.

How Liza confounded the experts and defied the odds is shared in her first book *Live Well with Chronic Pain,* where she chronicles the basic steps of her own recovery in an engaging storytelling style, explaining the "Four Foundations of Living Well with Chronic Pain." Now, in *Cupid's Challenge*, she takes on the task of teaching people how to achieve intimate pleasure and fulfillment in the face of chronic pain—a problem that affects literally millions of couples in the United States. She does not write just about refreshing your sexual relationship while managing chronic pain. But perhaps more importantly she writes about reconnecting, responding, and rejoicing in the physical and emotional intimacy that each relationship needs to flourish!

The book's path to re-engaging in pleasurable and sexual intimacy has two stages. The first chapters "set the stage," detailing some of the many ways chronic pain can interfere with and change couples' sex lives and intimacy. The second half of the book outlines focused, effective responses that can be playful, fun, sensuous, and emotionally bonding, leading to more fulfilling intimacy in the bedroom. Perhaps the most valuable feature of the book is that it provides partners with abundant hints and strategies that can help them to begin communicating about very delicate subjects. Liza's hope is that couples facing the challenge of chronic pain will be able to read and discuss *Cupid's Challenge* together, however many of its ideas can be put into practice even if only one member of the couple reads the book.

Throughout her writings, you will see aspects of Liza's patient-physician encounters. By infusing the voices and thoughts of these relationships with her own personal feelings and knowledge, she has succeeded in drawing universal lessons from those who suffer with chronic pain. When you read *Cupid's Challenge*, you will find it is positive, hopeful, and inspirational. In fact, Liza has issued an invitation to join her in learning how to regain much of the sexuality that you and your partner may feel you have lost as well as to accompany her on the path to becoming a THRIVER.

Before closing, I should explain why her book has special meaning for me. There are three reasons. First, I have known and worked with Liza for a number of years and am proud to have been her mentor, friend, and business partner during that time. Our friendship began during some of her darkest days in dealing with her own chronic pain, and it has been a pleasure to see her grow and thrive to the point that she is taking many of the lessons she has learned through her own personal challenges and in her medical practice to now share those insights with others.

The second reason is that this book stresses the importance of communication, respect, and appreciation in a relationship troubled by pain issues—I have found those to be keys for success in any relationship, business or personal. I know good communication to be absolutely imperative in working out issues, coming to successful conclusions, and solidifying relationships. It is important to understand that the person who loves the one in pain suffers also, because they hate seeing their loved one hurting and often feel helpless as well. As a result, I have seen patients come to realize that communication, loving respect and forgiveness are certainly important for couples beset by chronic pain who want to gain greater intimacy. In fact, even couples not troubled by chronic pain may find that Liza's words of wisdom help them invigorate the romance in their relationship.

And finally, the third reason is my own belief and interest in promoting health and a better quality of life for all of us, now and in the future. That includes promoting effective strategies to deal with pain issues, which at some point in our lives we may all face. Like Liza, I have seen how chronic pain can detrimentally affect many facets of people's lives. Since intimacy is one of the most important of these facets, I welcome a resource that can help couples successfully cope with the effects of pain in the bedroom. Liza and I are thus on a similar path. And because of my understanding of the serious effects of chronic pain, her book strikes me as a timely addition to the literature on health and good relationships. I trust you will see in it what I do—very positive, practical, and sound approaches to a problem that besets millions of people.

With that, I hope you will take the journey through *Cupid's Challenge*, engage your partner, and rekindle your relationship until the flames of passion and joy burn bright!

# Introduction

*Devastating.* There is no better word to summarize the effects of chronic pain on the lives of countless people. For months, years, even decades, recurring pain can impinge on virtually every aspect of daily life. Work, leisure, sleep, even the simplest pleasures can become casualties. According to a 2011 and 2014 Institute of Medicine report, over 100 million Americans experience chronic pain thus making that condition one of the nation's greatest enemies of wellbeing.

Fortunately, the prevalence of persistent pain in our society is starting to be recognized, and its many adverse consequences understood. Yet, one of its most widespread effects—the impact on sexual relationships—is seldom discussed. Even though chronic pain seriously disrupts the sex lives of millions of couples, far too little information is available and too much silence surrounds the topic.

This silence can often seem deafening in the bedrooms in which the problems arise. Taboos surrounding sexual intimacy and dysfunction frequently leave partners too embarrassed and vulnerable to talk about the issue. Instead of addressing their difficulty together, they may barely acknowledge it. As a result, the problem may worsen, often with serious repercussions in other areas of their relationship.

Are you and your partner facing such issues? Is one or both of you living with chronic pain that impinges on your sexual happiness? If so, this book can help you, in part because I am going to put aside taboos or embarrassment about the topics of chronic pain and sexual fulfillment. I am going to address forthrightly the issue that I call *Cupid's Challenge*—the problem of how partners can achieve a satisfying and intimate sexual relationship while coping with chronic pain. And I am going to explain how you and your lover can rise to the challenge by becoming Cupid's most powerful allies.

As a physician specializing in chronic pain, and a chronic pain survivor with rheumatoid arthritis myself, I know how pain interferes with sexual lives and how difficult it can be to address the problem. I have also come to understand how few resources are available to assist couples in dealing with these issues that strike at the core of their relationship.

So I decided to write a book with practical ideas that couples can use to address Cupid's Challenge in four dimensions: physically, psychologically, relationally, and sensually. Here, you will learn how to identify the ways in which the challenges arise for you and your partner. You will discover specific techniques and strategies that you can use to deal with the problem in all four dimensions. And you will learn how to design an effective multidimensional response that fits your specific situation.

An important theme that runs throughout this book is that people who deal with chronic pain are strong, often much stronger than they realize. Every day they face and overcome challenges beyond the ones experienced by others. For that reason, I call them not "sufferers," but *survivors*—survivors who just by doing their best every day living with persistent pain are, in my view, true champions.

They are so strong, in fact, they can become even more than survivors. They can become thrivers. Thrivers are people who grasp life firmly and strive for the fullest and best that they can achieve and enjoy. This, above all, is something that I love to see. By striving to live a fuller life, they are already living more fully. They are already thriving.

In my previous book, *Live Well with Chronic Pain: A Journey of Discovery,* I focused on that very thing—becoming a chronic pain thriver. My central theme was that those of us who live with chronic pain CAN live a full life. I talked briefly about sexual issues in relation to chronic pain. However, this crucial topic deserves its own treatment.

My main message here is that you and your partner CAN become chronic pain thrivers in the bedroom. You can assume an empowering attitude toward your pain and yourself. You can become more comfortable in your own skin, and feel romantic and sexy despite chronic pain. And you can turn the tables on pain to enjoy again the sexual happiness that is your natural right. Here, as in all aspects of your life, you CAN thrive even with chronic pain.

The fact that you have chosen this book and are actively seeking solutions to Cupid's Challenge is a great sign that you are already a thriver. My job is to provide you with important information and ideas that you can take with you into the bedroom to help you thrive even more.

I have divided the book into two main parts, with chapters one through three comprising part one. In chapter one I introduce you to why Cupid's Challenge is both important and complex. In chapter two, we will talk in detail about how chronic pain affects couples' sex lives in four important dimensions: physiological, psychological, relational, and sensual. This will help lay the groundwork for later chapters. In chapter three entitled "Getting Heat from *ICE*," you will learn a method that you and your partner can immediately put to work for you.

The second part of the book is where we start dealing with the specifics of Cupid's Challenge. It consists of nine chapters that address all four dimensions of the problem. In each chapter, I will focus on specific ideas that you and your partner can use to create a more fulfilling sexual relationship despite chronic pain. I also stay with the metaphor of Cupid's arrows. These arrows consist of various strategies that couples can use to address Cupid's Challenge—health, attitude, innovation, and many others. Just as Cupid's arrows are meant to bind lovers together, the ideas in each chapter are designed to help you and your partner join together more pleasurably as you solidify your sexual bond.

So let's get to it! The sooner we do, the sooner you can achieve your healthy and well-deserved rewards: closeness, sensuality, and scintillating sex.

# Chapter One

# *Cupid's Challenge*

## The Intruder

An uninvited and most unwelcome visitor is repeatedly showing up in the bedrooms of millions of couples. This visitor often arrives at the most inopportune time—just as the lovers are turning to one another to enjoy the sensuous pleasures that are their natural right. At that special moment, the visitor—I should say trespasser—brashly bangs through the bedroom door, forcing its way into their embrace.

Often, the intruder doesn't even wait that long. It may sneak into the room with the couple as they prepare for bed, not allowing them time to get comfortable or to touch each other, before causing dismay and disruption. And then, despite the partners' great desire that the interloper go away and leave them alone, it stays, making it difficult for them to enjoy even a few minutes of the sweet erotic pleasures that they once took for granted.

This obnoxious intruder I am referring to, the one who moves into the sanctity of countless couples' bedrooms, is chronic pain. By chronic pain, I mean pain that frequently occurs over a period of months or years. Such pain is usually associated with a specific condition or disability such as arthritis, low back strain, nerve injury, recurrent headaches, and many other conditions. The Institute of Medicine's findings revealing that there are more than one hundred million Americans who suffer from some form of chronic pain only tells part of the story though as there are no precise statistics on how many of these people are married or are otherwise committed to one another. However, in the United States alone, the institute's same report suggests that likely tens of millions of couples have at least one partner who lives with recurrent pain arising from some persistent ailment.

Dealing with chronic pain can negatively affect couples' lives in many ways. It may, for example, have profound effects on one or both partners' occupational goals and other dreams for the future. Or it may adversely affect the couple's finances, leisure-time activities, or ability to enjoy the company of their children, relatives, and friends. There is no end to the ways in which chronic pain can cause serious problems in people's lives.

One of the most frustrating ways is when pain creates sexual difficulties by invading the bedroom. Repeated outbreaks of pain often interfere with, complicate, and detract from sexual relationships. And in many cases, they virtually devastate the couple's love life.

If you, your partner, or both of you are among the millions living with chronic pain, the metaphorical picture I drew of what it's like when pain encroaches on the bedroom may have evoked a nod of recognition. That picture was a general one, but there are a multitude of very specific ways in which recurrent pain may be interfering with your sex life. Some of the most common include:

- Conditions such as arthritis and low back problems cause decreased flexibility and an inhibited range of motion for one or more parts of the body. The afflicted individual may have to be cautious in positioning and moving their limbs, torso, neck, or head. This may place substantial restrictions on the activities in bed.
- Other ailments result in ultrasensitive skin that can erupt in pain if touched without great care, or even if touched at all. Because sex requires bodily contact, this can seriously inhibit sensual activities.
- Temporomandibular joint dysfunction (commonly known as TMJ), a syndrome that often results in severe pain in the jaw, can restrict individuals' ability to enjoy oral sex.

- Other painful conditions, such as chronic headaches or recurrent gastrointestinal pain, can cause severe discomfort and significantly inhibit sexual activity.

The particular ways in which these or other conditions affect a couple's sex life will of course depend on the specifics of the ailment. However, it's often not so much the underlying condition that hinders enjoyable sex, but rather the pain that accompanies it. One woman expressed this to me in the following way: "It's not my arthritis per se that makes sex such a huge problem—it's the pain it causes. If I could just get rid of that pain, then, stiff or not, I'm sure my husband and I could enjoy sex again."

It's easy to understand this woman's thought because we are all familiar with how pain overcomes our senses. The basic way is by being an acute experience that commands our attention. In doing so, it counteracts sensations of pleasure that we might otherwise enjoy. Sexual delight is rooted in sensuality which involves pleasurable feelings, while painful sensations tend to overwhelm these finer feelings. Thus, sensual pleasures become lost in the excruciating sensations of pain in the way that a beautiful song playing might get lost in the sound of a jackhammer churning outside your window.

Having sexual relations may even exacerbate the pain. The afflicted partner's discomfort may increase because the couple is using positions or techniques that aggravate the painful area. As a result, both partners enjoy sex less when they do engage in it, and as a result over time they will likely find themselves reducing their sexual activity even more.

## The Many Values of Sex
You know Cupid—that naked, curly-headed baby boy we tend to see a lot of around Valentine's Day. Actually, Cupid is the ancient Roman god of erotic love. His modern-day job is to fly around with his bow and arrows, bringing lovers' hearts and bodies together to join in sensuous, ecstatic embraces.

Cupid's job is crucial because erotic love—sex—is such an important part of the lives of most adult couples. In fact, it would be pretty hard to overestimate the significance of sex. Its importance begins with the essential role it plays in procreation. Through the sexual union of men and women, the human race succeeds, generation after generation, in extending its existence.

However, reproduction isn't the only value of sex, not by any means. Consider this:

Sex is one of the main motivators behind human behavior. To ensure the survival of the species, the biological drive that urges lovers to mate has to be powerful. One result is that much of the behavior of many, if not most, young adults is focused on locating, courting, and keeping a suitable mate. And it's not just younger folks who are strongly influenced by sexual objectives. Sex is a prime motivator for adults of all ages.

Erotic love is one of the great pleasures of life. To make sure we won't neglect our duty to promulgate, nature has designed us to be sensual creatures who are capable of enjoying exquisite physical pleasure while engaging in sexual activity. The experience of a powerful orgasm is the most focused form of this pleasure; however, sexual enjoyment can take other forms. In fact, many couples find great pleasure simply in mutual touching, or in cuddling and holding one another.

Sex draws couples closer together. Sex is clearly physical, but it is often emotional as well. Lovers reveal their naked bodies to one another and join together to provide mutual pleasure that can lead these engagements to often generate a degree of intimacy that no other relationship can offer. So it is understandable that the one individual in the world who we typically feel closest to is our partner.

Sex is fulfilling. The fact that we humans are sexual beings means that we find self-fulfillment through expressing our sexuality in appropriate ways. When erotic love has an unsatisfactory place within a couple's life, they may feel that an important part of their inner self is not being realized. And no wonder. By not fully experiencing the pleasure and intimacy of sexual union, they are missing out on potential joy from their relationship.

---

**Cupid's Point**

In each chapter, I am going to insert several boxed entries that I call *Cupid's Points.* Their purpose is to encourage you to focus on how the issues being discussed arise in your life. So, here's your first Cupid's Point:

Did you notice that the values of erotic love listed are interconnected? For example, increased physical pleasure from sex often binds partners more tightly together emotionally. Now ask yourself: In what ways are the different values of sex connected in your own love life? Which of these values are most important to you? To your partner?

---

From all of this, it's evident that Cupid is not just an antiquated Roman myth whose only role is to decorate Valentine's Day cards. He is a very active player in the happiest and healthiest intimate relationships using his bow and arrows to bind partners together in an embrace of sexual love.

And this is true for couples of all ages. There is a widespread misconception that erotic love is only for young or middle-aged couples, and that it's rarely enjoyed by older ones. However, although sexual desire typically wanes to some extent as individuals age and relationships mature, it seldom disappears completely. Often, Cupid is still prominent in the lives of more seasoned partners. I know couples in their eighties and older who enjoy an active sex life that gives them great delight. And their satisfaction arises for the same reasons that younger couples enjoy sex—because it feels good physically, binds the partners together emotionally, and creates a greater sense of fulfillment in their lives.

## Cupid's Challenge and this Book

With all of the important benefits that erotic love has going for it, you might think that Cupid's job would be a relatively simple one. But by striking at the core of sensuality, which is the basis of sex, chronic pain can cause Cupid's arrows of connection to go wildly astray. In fact, chronic pain creates one of Cupid's greatest challenges. Essentially, this great challenge—which I naturally call *Cupid's Challenge*—can be put in the form of a question:

*How can partners achieve a happy and fulfilling sex life when one or both are living with chronic pain?*

For millions of couples, this is an issue of profound importance because of the immense value that enjoying a fulfilling sex life offers. I am going to assume that it's also an important issue for you.

But even if you are in a partnership not currently facing Cupid's Challenge however are living with chronic pain, or you may be single now and experiencing chronic pain but are contemplating entering into a relationship, or perhaps you have recently begun a relationship and are unsure about whether your or your partner's painful condition might result in sexual difficulties, in all of these cases, the approaches suggested here may still prove to be valuable to you in the future.

Even in a case where your partner doesn't want to talk about the Cupid's Challenge you may be experiencing, you may still find here useful strategies that will help improve the communication between you or that can otherwise be applied to improve the situation in your bedroom. As you will discover, I have designed these tools for a wide range of scenarios in which Cupid's Challenge may arise in your life.

## Cupid's Challenge Has Many Aspects

In addition to the two basic problems that I described earlier—that pain tends to overwhelm sensuality and that engaging in sex may make pain worse—I have also found in my practice that pain often seriously detracts from partners' sex lives in subtle, yet powerful ways that they may not fully recognize.

This is illustrated by a situation for a couple in their late thirties trying to cope with the effects of chronic pain in their bedroom. Bonnie was a patient of mine who was suffering from systematic lupus erythematosus, better known simply as lupus or SLE, an autoimmune disease that typically results in arthritis-like symptoms, including swollen joints, while her husband Ned was growing increasingly sexually frustrated.

## Bonnie and Ned's Story

*Bonnie was on medications that usually kept her pain at a tolerable level, but on one of her visits with me she revealed that she and Ned had recently begun experiencing some sexual difficulties due to pain arising from her condition. She told me that when they engaged in sex, which had been about twice a week during most of the past year, they tried to be very careful to reduce pressure on any of her sensitive joints. Even so, pain occasionally erupted if inadvertent stress was placed on a knee, wrist, or elbow. When that occurred, Bonnie invariably called a halt to their intimacy. Even if the flare-up lasted for only a few seconds, and Ned suggested changing their position to alleviate the stress, Bonnie made it clear she was out of the mood and would prefer to go to sleep.*

*Such a turn of events always left Ned frustrated, Bonnie told me. He showed it by lying awake afterward, silent but obviously perturbed, while Bonnie tried to sleep. In time, his frustration had taken a toll on him. Over the next few months, he approached Bonnie for sex less often. And even when she instigated the encounter, he sometimes declined. At the time of our conversation, the couple's lovemaking had slowed to where they engaged in sex only two or three times a month. Even on that reduced schedule, pain would still sometimes strike Bonnie and interrupt their time together.*

*In describing the situation, Bonnie expressed a lack of understanding about what was happening to her and Ned. She had little insight into their problem, so I suggested what is always an excellent idea if couples are facing issues of any kind—communication. I urged her to engage Ned in an honest discussion so that the two of them could come to a better understanding of their problem.*

*When I saw Bonnie six weeks later, I was pleased to learn that she had taken my advice. She and Ned had enjoyed several frank discussions about their changed sex life and had discovered things about each other and themselves that they had not realized. For instance, Bonnie found out that the reason Ned had become less interested in sex was that he felt rejected when she "shut him down" after she had an episode of pain. He hated the feeling of being rejected.*

*During their talks, Bonnie also discovered something important about her own feelings—that the main reason she refused to go any further after a pain flare-up was that it caused her to feel embarrassed and unattractive. She even felt that by calling a halt to their intimacy, she was somehow doing Ned a favor. "I thought he wouldn't have to waste his time trying to make love to such a pathetic crybaby," she said.*

*When Ned learned of her feelings, he insisted that he had never felt that way about her. He again emphasized that his problem had been his sense of feeling rejected.*

*Bonnie happily shared with me that their new understandings had made an immense difference in their sex life. Now, if she started feeling pain while they were having sex, she rested for a few minutes while Ned gently stroked her and talked about how much he wanted to make love to her—which she found to be very erotic. If the pain persisted, they would agree to try again soon. In most cases, however, they were able to continue and enjoy their time together. As a result, their overall sexual enjoyment became greater than it had been for years.*

What Bonnie and Ned's story illustrates—aside from the crucial importance of communication—is that chronic pain can also create many other negative consequences that a couple might be unaware of. Here are some examples of these and how they can interfere with a couple's sexual happiness:

Having to deal with chronic pain can generate negative feelings that inhibit sexual pleasure and fulfillment. Good sex goes hand in hand with positive feelings of mental relaxation, sensuality, companionship, and lightness. Chronic pain though may radically interfere with such positive emotions by generating feelings of irritation, anxiety, anger, or even hopelessness.

Persistent pain can negatively affect self-image, causing the person to feel over-the-hill or otherwise unsexy. Repeated experiences of severe pain can lead the affected individual to feel debilitated. From there, it doesn't take much to start thinking, "I'm not who I used to be. I just don't have it any more." The individual may become further convinced that he or she is no longer attractive, or even no longer a sexual being.

Being afflicted with chronic pain and its sexual effects can lead a person to feel embarrassed or guilty. Individuals dealing with chronic pain may feel embarrassed about the need to be careful in bed, or feel guilty about their condition believing that they are placing a burden on their partner. Such feelings can raise anxieties that hinder the coming together of lovers in a mutually satisfying sexual union. Instead, the afflicted individual may lean in the opposite direction and try to avoid sexual situations.

Dealing with chronic pain can consume a great deal of energy, making the individual too weary for sex. The energy consumed may be both physical and psychological. Anyone who has suffered through a prolonged episode consisting of a severe headache, toothache, strained back, or other painful event knows that the experience tends to be both physically demanding and mentally wearing. This is all the more true when the painful events occur repeatedly. The end result is that a painful episode can leave the individual with less physical and psychic energy to expend on sexual activity and he or she may just want to rest or go to sleep.

Some pain medications can decrease libido. This is a "Catch-22" factor. The medicine that helps make it possible to experience pain-free sex may have the unfortunate side effect of decreasing the person's desire for intimate activity. This kind of situation is one variant of the more general problem of medications that are effective in one area but may reduce quality of life in another.

Chronic pain may place strains on other aspects of a couple's relationship, and these may adversely affect their sex life. Such aspects may include finances, careers, care of children, and other central elements of the couple's life together. For example, if chronic pain leads to difficulties in securing or retaining a job, which in turn leads to financial problems, the resulting stress and worry may result in one or both partners having decreased desire for sexual relations.

Even when pain is not present, the knowledge that it might arise at any moment can inhibit sexual pleasure and fulfillment. This can happen in several ways. For example, the fear that pain may suddenly arise can cause anxiety in one or both partners to a degree that it decreases the couple's pleasure when they do have sex. Or, it may cause them to rush through their sexual engagement as they try to make sure they are complete before the pain comes back. In either case, pain succeeds in reaching out its ghostly hand even when it's not actually present to inhibit the couple's love life.

---

Cupid's Point

Did any of the kinds of problems described seem to be relevant to Bonnie and Ned's sex life before they started communicating? Which one(s)?

Do any of those kinds of problems arise for you or your partner? If so, which do you think most seriously affect your sex life? Are any of the problems related to one another?

---

## Becoming Cupid's Indispensable Assistants

"But what can I do to make things better? Pain is pain, right? And when it's having its way with me, what is there to do but take a pill and wait it out?" I sometimes hear comments like these in regards to coping with chronic pain. The words express the idea that because pain is a physiological matter, there's not much that can be done about it—or its effects—except get the latest prescription and try not to aggravate the condition that gives rise to the pain.

I strongly disagree with that attitude. Individuals living with chronic pain can almost always do a great deal to cope with the effects of their condition. And that includes making a difference in the way pain affects their sexual activities. Bonnie and Ned proved that fact to themselves by coming to a better understanding of how pain was impinging on their sex life and then changing their behavior accordingly.

You and your partner can do the same. The particular ways in which Cupid's Challenge arises in your lives and how you can best address the challenge may likely to be different from Bonnie and Ned's situation. But the idea that there is nothing to be done is, to use an old-fashioned word, hogwash.

There is actually much you can do to address the way chronic pain affects your sex life. You don't have to respond to the challenge haphazardly or throw up your hands in defeat. For example, you can develop a focused and effective response by using strategies and ideas that you discover in this book. Though you may need to make some changes in how you go about things, many tools here can help you and your lover enjoy greater sexual pleasure and intimacy while managing chronic pain.

When you employ those tools, you will be acting as Cupid's indispensable assistants, helping him to get your love life on track. After all, who's going to get that job done if not you? You are the ones who must sharpen Cupid's arrows and guide his eye and hands to make sure those arrows are launched with accuracy.

---

Cupid's Point

If you are living with chronic pain, how would you describe your general attitude toward that fact? Do you take an active part in managing your condition and your pain?

How does your and your partner's attitudes, positive or negative, currently affect the way pain impacts your sex life?

---

## Scintillating Sex

What Cupid wants for you and your partner, and what you likely want to aim for, is *scintillating* sex. By using that term, I'm not referring to a sex life that's super "steamy," or to some other feature that's supposed to pertain to every couple's sexual activities. It would be silly to try to name such a characteristic because every couple, being composed of two unique people, is itself unique. What makes for a happy, satisfying, and fulfilling sexual relationship for each couple will depend on their particular desires and ways of relating to one another.

Instead, scintillating sex is something that's defined by the couple themselves. For young newlyweds and some others, scintillating sex may consist of frequent multi-orgasmic encounters that leave both lovers thoroughly exhausted and satiated. For the mature couple, gentle touching, holding, and cuddling within a context of intimacy and loving acceptance may provide great emotional and physical pleasure. Both kinds of activity, along with everything in between, can count as great sex depending on the couple's desires and needs. Scintillating sex, in other words, is simply what satisfies you and your partner.

And that's wonderful, because it means you and your partner don't have to meet an external standard of sexual performance or pleasure in order to achieve scintillating sex. Cupid doesn't want you to live by someone else's rules. He wants the two of you to understand what's right for you sexually, and then to achieve your sexual happiness together in your own way.

There is only one quality that pertains to scintillating sex for every couple. It's not a particular kind of activity or way of doing things. But rather it's that the best sex always occurs when partners are on the same wavelength in their enjoyment of each other. That's often something that couples who are dealing with chronic pain (as well as many other couples) are lacking. And it's all the more reason for you and your partner to deal with Cupid's Challenge *together.*

Remember that *scintillating* sex is simply pleasurable, fulfilling, and happy sex. You and your partner are the only ones to determine what that is for the two of you. And the ones to then go for it!

# Chapter Two

# Meeting Cupid's Challenge with Many Arrows

Arthritis, lupus, back strains, neck problems, migraines—every condition gives rise to its own kind of distress. When you add the fact that every relationship is unique, it's easy to see why chronic pain can affect couples' sexual relations in countless ways.

However, there is a general approach that couples can use to meet Cupid's Challenge. In this chapter I am going to explain a general way of dealing with Cupid's Challenge that makes good sense whether the pain affecting your relationship arises from osteoarthritis, endometriosis, stress headaches, a slipped disc, or some other ailment.

## The Multidimensional Approach

In looking for a general way to deal with Cupid's Challenge, the first idea that may occur is to take a purely physiological approach. At first glance, this seems reasonable. After all, pain is a physiological response to a physiological condition, and sex is a body-centered activity. However, we would be seriously limiting ourselves if we were to only follow this path to address Cupid's Challenge. For instance, we would be forgetting something that we touched on in chapter one—the fact that both chronic pain and sexuality extend far beyond the body in their connections and meanings. They also involve partners' thoughts and judgments, attitudes and emotions, and many aspects of how the couple relates to one another.

This was recently brought home to me again while I was giving a talk to a group of chronic pain survivors about the effects of pain on relationships. During the discussion period afterward, an attractive, well-dressed woman of about forty—I'll call her Karen—shared with the group that after being divorced for several years, she was lonely and often thought about entering into a new relationship. But she had serious doubts about doing so due to the rheumatoid arthritis that had begun afflicting her. She especially had qualms about engaging in sexual activity.

I asked whether her concern was about how pain might arise during sexual encounters. She replied that she thought that if she was careful, most of the pain could be avoided. What really bothered her though was the fact that she would have to be somewhat cautious during sex, because she didn't think that anyone would find her attractive if she had to "tiptoe around" in bed.

Karen's words clearly illustrated how chronic pain often affects sexual relations on more than just the physiological level. For her, Cupid's Challenge took on the form of hesitancy about entering into a sexual relationship. But her hesitancy had more to do with her *attitude* toward her pain and managing it during sex than it did with the pain itself. Which means there is a strong psychological element in the way that Cupid's Challenge arises for her.

Here are some other ways that chronic pain and sexuality go far beyond the purely physical:

- Whatever emotions we experience during sex—from love to anxiety, from anger to joy—affect our sexual satisfaction.
- Our mental states help to determine how well we manage our chronic pain. They even affect the way we experience pain.
- What we think about ourself, our body, and our partner has a profound effect on our sexual enjoyment.
- A partner's strong support can help a chronic pain survivor become a thriver.

- Good communication between partners is crucial for understanding how chronic pain may be affecting their sex life and what they can do about it.

In these and many other ways, chronic pain and sexuality are interwoven physiologically, psychologically, sensually, and relationally in partnerships. In fact, we would be hard-pressed to find any two segments of our lives that more fully engage our physical, mental, and social selves than do chronic pain and sexuality.

These considerations indicate that to truly address Cupid's Challenge, we need to understand all these important ways that chronic pain may intersect with our sexual lives, and then seek strategies that can help us deal with the problem with this global thinking. In a word, we should take a *multidimensional* approach to Cupid's Challenge.

A multidimensional approach to an issue is one that considers a variety of dimensions or aspects. Such an approach is often necessary when dealing with human problems because we are such wonderfully complex, many-sided creatures. And that's exactly what we need to do with Cupid's Challenge.

The word *multidimensional* also connotes the idea of depth. In art, a three-dimensional rendering of a scene adds perspective and depth that can't be captured in a two-dimensional representation. Similarly, a multidimensional understanding of how chronic pain can undermine sexual relations adds new perspectives, insights, and depths that are lost if we restrict ourselves to only a single dimension.

### The Four Dimensions of Cupid's Challenge

The value of a multidimensional approach to Cupid's Challenge becomes even more evident when we examine particular cases in which chronic pain is wreaking havoc on a couple's sex life. For instance, consider the plight of Howard and Barbara, a couple in their fifties, both on their second marriage. When I first met them, they reported that for most of their five years together their sex life was good. But over the past several months, things had changed considerably. By looking carefully at the couple's situation, we will find validation for the multidimensional approach. We will also discover just how many dimensions Cupid's Challenge can involve.

<u>Howard and Barbara's Story</u>

*Howard sat in his easy chair, his lower back supported by a small cushion, as he watched the Sunday night football game. It was ten thirty, time for bed, but the contest was only in the third quarter.*

*Howard was secretly glad the game was far from over. Not because it was a particularly exciting match or because one of his favorite teams was playing. In fact, he didn't care much about who won the game. But it did give him an excuse to not go to bed soon.*

*He heard Barbara come out of the bath and stop at the door to the bedroom. He pretended to be engrossed in the TV.*

*After a moment she said, "Are you coming to bed, Dear?"*

*Howard turned to his wife. "Hon, I think I'll stay up a bit longer to watch a little more of this game. It's a pretty good matchup tonight. I'll just watch for another fifteen or twenty minutes."*

*"How's your back?"*

*A brief scowl erupted on his face. "It's fine," he said. "Never felt better."*

*"All right then, I'll keep the bed warm for you."*

*"Thanks, Hon," replied Howard, forcing a smile. "I'll be there soon."*

*Once Barbara had closed the bedroom door, he sat gazing at the TV but not really watching the game. He suddenly felt dejected and cowardly. Lying to his wife to avoid situations where she might expect intimacy was becoming a habit, he realized, and he didn't like himself for it.*

*But what else can I do? he thought. It was the fault of that low back pain that had been nagging him since he strained it a few months before in June. Though he had become increasingly careful in his activities since then, he never seemed to have a pain-free day anymore. Despite what he had said to Barbara, even now he could feel the pain tentatively edging along his lower spine. He carefully adjusted the cushion, but it didn't help much.*

If it hurts just from sitting here doing nothing, *he thought,* God only knows how much it would be bothering me if I were in the bedroom trying to be a stud! *He remembered the last time he had attempted to make love with Barbara. When was that—three weeks ago? What a fiasco that had been. The back spasm had struck less than a moment after they started having intercourse. How embarrassing!*

*And it wasn't just the back pain. A few months ago he had begun having occasional difficulty in keeping an erection—something that had never happened to him before. Thank goodness he had somehow managed to keep the fact from Barbara. At least he hoped he had. He had thought briefly about seeing his doctor about the problem, and maybe asking if those pills meant to deal with that kind of problem might work for him too. But the idea of taking a pill to give himself an erection ... well, that just didn't sound very manly to him.*

*What a change all this represented. For the previous four and half years of their marriage, their sex life had been just right. But not anymore.* Let's face it, Howard, *he thought glumly.* You're almost over-the-hill. *It was a thought that he had begun repeating often in his mind.*

*In the meantime, Barbara lay in the darkened bedroom wondering if her husband was truly interested in the football game. She thought about how almost every night now they seemed to go to bed at different times. Or if they went to bed together, Howard would immediately announce how tired he was, making it clear that he was not interested in any sexual activity.*

I don't understand what's happening to us, *she thought.* Am I that unattractive? Or does it have something to do with his back? He seldom complains about it these days, but I know it still bothers him. He saw the doctor shortly after he sprained it, but he hasn't gone back. If he would make another appointment, perhaps the doctor could prescribe something that would help. Maybe I should mention it, but I would hate for him to think I was nagging him.

*She listened to the murmur of the television in the next room, wishing that the noise would end and Howard would appear at the bedroom door.* But I know he won't be to bed until much later, *she thought as she lay there feeling helpless. She just didn't know what to do.*

The difficult issues illustrated by this account are all too common among couples who face Cupid's Challenge. What makes the story especially heartbreaking is the way the partners handled their problem. Or perhaps I should say, *did not* handle it. Unfortunately, this—the failure of couples to come to grips with their difficulties—is something I see far too often.

Howard and Barbara's story provides a clear illustration of how their situation incorporates four main dimensions.

### The Physiological Dimension

This aspect of Howard and Barbara's problem is most obviously represented by Howard's back condition and its attendant pain. A related physiological fact is that he has not consulted a physician about the back condition except for one visit that he made soon after it began. We know that he sometimes self-treats by using a pillow to support his back when he sits. But he appears to have made little systematic effort to deal with the problem, which indicates that he is not taking full ownership of his condition.

The physiological dimension is also represented by the fact that Howard has experienced some difficulty maintaining an erection during the past few months. This is making him even more hesitant to engage in sex. It is also possible that his erection difficulties are being exacerbated by his chronic pain. But here, too, he has been reluctant to consult a physician about the problem, which prevents him from dealing with it effectively.

### The Psychological Dimension

This aspect occurs in the couple's situation in several important ways. For one thing, Howard feels embarrassed at having gotten a back spasm the last time he attempted to have intercourse with his wife. Fear of that happening again is now making him reluctant to engage in sex at all. He is also embarrassed about his occasional erectile dysfunction, which is probably adding to his fear of failure.

In addition, Howard seems to have a self-defeating perspective about his sexuality, one that isn't helping him deal effectively with the situation. For instance, he often thinks that his back pain and occasional erection difficulties show that he is "over-the-hill," which suggests that he views both conditions as detracting from his masculinity. As for the erectile difficulty, he believes that taking an erection-enhancing drug would not be a "manly" thing to do.

Yet another aspect of the psychological dimension for Howard is that there doesn't seem to be a lot of fight in him in regard to dealing with the problem. That's not to say he is content with what's happening, for he obviously feels guilt and anxiety about it. But he seems to think that he's helpless to do anything much to remedy the situation.

An attitude of helplessness is also Barbara's main response. She isn't even sure whether it's Howard's pain that's leading him to be less interested in sex, or something else. Though she thinks briefly about suggesting to Howard that he see his physician about his back, she's afraid that if she did so, he might think she was nagging him. The last thought she has before she drops off to sleep is that there is nothing she can do but hope for the best, which sounds like she is giving up.

## The Relational Dimension

This aspect encompasses how Howard and Barbara relate to and communicate with one another. It includes Howard's recent behavior of either avoiding going to bed at the same time as Barbara, or immediately announcing that he is tired. These behaviors mark a radical change in a sex life that had previously been satisfying for both partners.

This relationship dimension also includes the important repercussion that in trying to avoid sexual activity, Howard often lies to

Barbara. He tells her he wants to watch football when what he actually wants to do is avoid sex. In bed, when he says he's tired, it's just an act, one that he puts on to dampen any expectation of sexual activity.

Howard also has other secrets that he keeps from his wife. He doesn't want Barbara to know about his erectile difficulty because it embarrasses him. And he seems to want to downplay his back pain to Barbara. Perhaps he thinks that communicating clearly about his pain would also not be "manly."

But Barbara isn't the world's best communicator either. She seems hesitant to dig below the surface to understand why Howard hasn't been interested in sex lately. Whatever the reason, she isn't proactive in trying to uncover the truth about his back pain and his reasons for avoiding sex.

Evidently, Howard and Barbara's lack of forthright communication is a main roadblock to their being able to deal effectively with their problems in bed. In fact, it's hard to see how they can even understand the problem, let alone deal with it, unless they start communicating.

In sum, each of these three dimensions plays a crucial role in how Cupid's Challenge manifests itself in this couple's lives:

- The physiological dimension is expressed by Howard's chronic pain, his occasional erection problems, and his failure to vigorously pursue medical help for either condition.
- The psychological dimension is present in both partners' thoughts, judgments, feelings, and attitudes about what is happening.
- The relational dimension is represented by the couple's deteriorating sexual relations and their lack of communication about their problem.

In addition to these three, there is a fourth dimension of the couple's situation. This aspect may not be obvious at first, but once recognized, it's evident that it can be of immense importance for understanding and dealing with Cupid's Challenge.

## The Sensual Dimension

This aspect of Howard and Barbara's situation encompasses their actual behavior in their sexual encounters—what kinds of things they tend to do, as well as when, where, and how they do them. It also includes their *sensual savvy,* which encompasses what they know about various ways to achieve sensual enjoyment in their relationship. More specifically, their sensual savvy refers to: How much do Howard and Barbara know about what pleases themselves and each other? How skilled are they in sensually pleasing each other? Have they investigated any new ways in which they might increase their sexual pleasure while minimizing Howard's pain?

---

Cupid's Point

One good way to start increasing your *sensual savvy* is to ask yourself a few questions. For example:

- Do your sexual encounters always follow the same general pattern?
- Do you ever wish to try something new with your partner?
- If so, might these new ways of relating reduce the effect of chronic pain on your sexual relations?
- Do you ever tell your mate what you would like to try?

Ask your partner to answer these same questions. Compare answers and use them as a springboard to discussion—which could end up being a very sexy one.

---

The evidence suggests that this couple's—or at least Howard's—sensual savvy is pretty low. For one thing, Howard's main reason for avoiding sexual relations with Barbara is his fear that his back will start acting up during intercourse. This suggests that his idea of having sex doesn't go much beyond the thought of having intercourse. As he sits there feeling dejected about lying to his wife, he doesn't consider the possibility of joining her in some other pleasurable sexual activities that would put minimal strain on his back. Such activities might include sensually exploring each other's bodies with erotic touch, engaging in oral sex, or simply cuddling and holding each other.

Another indication that Howard's sensual savvy is low is that he assumes intercourse would likely cause his back pain to intensify. He doesn't seem to be aware that there are positions for intercourse that could result in very little strain to his back, thereby greatly reducing the possibility of a pain flare-up. Here too, one of the most effective things that Howard and Barbara could do to improve their sexual relations would be to develop their sensual savvy.

Overall, their sexual problems involve four key dimensions. In this, they are like millions of other couples who must cope with the effects of chronic pain on their sex life. Every situation is unique and how the dimensions interrelate will differ from couple to couple; but all four dimensions will almost always be present whenever a couple is facing Cupid's Challenge.

Therefore, if we want to deal comprehensively with Cupid's Challenge, we must learn strategies that address the challenge as it arises in each dimension. Strategies to increase sensual savvy may be right for some, while a physiological approach may be most useful for others. But virtually all couples coping with Cupid's Challenge will find some degree of attention is needed for every dimension.

## Think Multidimensionally

One of your main objectives here is to discover how the various dimensions relate to your situation. This means recognizing the way that chronic pain is affecting your relationship in the light of all four dimensions—physiological, psychological, relational, and sensual. Doing this will allow you to get the most comprehensive understanding of how Cupid's Challenge affects you and your partner. You will then be able to put what you learn to work by tailoring a multidimensional response to the challenge as it occurs.

Here are four specific actions that can help you gain a broader multidimensional view of your situation:

Write Down Your Story. Take a few minutes now to write out a personal account of how chronic pain is affecting your sexual relations. Your personal account may be short or long. You may write it jointly with your partner, or on your own. It may be in story form, or it could simply be a list of points that capture the main aspects of how your sex life is being disrupted by chronic pain. In any event, your personal account will help you to focus on Cupid's Challenge.

---

### Cupid's Point

Here are a few things to think about as you write your account of how Cupid's Challenge arises for you and your partner:

- How is each of the four dimensions represented in the way chronic pain affects your sexual relationship? Use Howard and Barbara's story as a model.
- Which dimensions seem most important in your situation?
- Think of three ways that different dimensions are interrelated for you and your partner.
- Is there one dimension that you believe you and your partner should focus on first? Or most?

---

As you work through this book, consult your account often. And as you read each chapter and come across new ideas and strategies, feel free to amend the account by adding further details. Or you may want to make a note on your account in the appropriate place when you come across a strategy that you think may be useful. Using your personal account in this way can help you keep focused on how various ideas and strategies for different dimensions may apply to you and your partner.

Look for Connections. As you work through the book and come across different dimensions, think about your situation in terms of possible connections between these dimensions and potential strategies to address your needs. For example, are aspects of communication (the relational dimension) affecting the degree of pain experienced by you or your partner? Is the degree of pain affecting communication? How is your and your partner's attitude affecting communication, pain, or willingness to increase sensual savvy?

Discovering connections can help you to uncover new realizations about the various factors affecting your circumstance. This, in turn, can help you to achieve a clearer and deeper understanding of how Cupid's Challenge arises for you and your partner. As you seek new connections, keep your written account close at hand and add to it as you wish.

Design a Multidimensional Strategy That Fits You. Recognizing connections between the different dimensions and individual strategies can help you design an effective multidimensional strategy to address Cupid's Challenge. This will not be a strategy that someone hands you already made, but one that you devise based on your knowledge of your own situation and on what you learn in this book. It will be a strategy specifically designed by you and your partner to fit *your* lives.

Look for Real, Not Necessarily Easy Solutions. Many of the strategies that you'll learn about will take work, dedication, and commitment. But don't let that scare you away. Look for real solutions, not necessarily easy ones. Good sex is such an important part of a fulfilling partnership that it's well worth the work required. And anyway, much of that "work" can be very enjoyable.

Sometimes a strategy may be relatively easy to enact. Remember Howard? If he would have just gotten out of that chair, gone into the bedroom, laid down with Barbara, held her, and said, "Hon, there's something I've been meaning to talk with you about." What a great way that would have been for him to start addressing Cupid's Challenge.

But if you or I were Howard, stuck in a certain way of viewing our situation, that might not be easy to do. That's another reason why writing an account of how chronic pain is affecting your sex life can be helpful. It requires you to stand outside the problem, which may enable you to more clearly see how to start dealing with it.

# Chapter Three

## Getting Heat From Ice

I hope that as you make your way through these chapters, you will regularly reread a section or two, pause to consider its ideas, then ask yourself a few practical questions such as:

- How do these ideas apply to my situation?
- How can they help me and my partner enjoy a more satisfying sex life?
- What can I do, and what can we do as a couple, to make the ideas work for us?

It is best if you and your partner read this book to each other at the breakfast table; or share ideas from it on a Sunday afternoon out on the patio; or the two of you read and talk about in bed as you lie close to one another.

In brief, I hope *Cupid's Challenge* will serve as a workbook. To make it so, you will need to do two things: read it carefully to locate the strategies that speak most directly to your situation, then commit yourselves to acting on those ideas. I believe that if you do that—if you work with the book—then the book will work for you.

### The *ICE* Method

To make this into a workbook, it will help if you have a method for translating the ideas on the page into action. In this chapter, I am going to explain such a method. It consists of three simple steps. By following them, you can prevent *Cupid's Challenge* from becoming a dust-gatherer that's full of promising ideas, though ones you never act upon.

The name of the method is *ICE,* which is an acronym for the three steps that comprise it—*Identify, Choose,* and *Explore.* These are three fairly distinct activities that can structure your efforts as you address Cupid's Challenge. By following them, you will be able to lift the book's ideas and techniques out of the realm of theory and into the reality of your life.

It will be helpful if after you read in later chapters more about the *Identify, Choose,* and *Explore* steps that you then circle back *to this point and re-read the explanations here to better fully understand the* whole method.

### The First Stage of *ICE*—*Identify*

The initial step of the *ICE* method—*Identify*—is based on the idea that to deal with a problem effectively, we need to understand what the problem is. So the better you understand the specific ways pain adversely affects your sex life, the more equipped you will be to apply helpful strategies.

Sounds easy, doesn't it? After all, aren't the negative effects of pain always pretty obvious? Actually, no. For many couples, identifying the ways that pain limits their sex life is not a simple task for a number of reasons.

First, the partners may not have a good understanding of the nature of the pain that is being experienced. For example, the one who actually feels the pain may have never clearly explained to their partner just what hurts, how much, and when. As a result, their lover may have only a vague grasp of what the problem is. Even the one suffering may have little understanding of the details beyond the fact that "it hurts!"

This points out the need for partners to identify, specifically, the character of the pain and its physiological effects. To do this, they should ask some basic questions to help them focus on the physiological nature of the problem. Questions such as:

- What part(s) of my (or my partner's) body hurts when we try to make love? Left knee? Neck? Specific areas of skin? The one with chronic pain should be as precise as possible when identifying those areas and sharing the information with their partner.

- At what point during lovemaking does the pain start or become too much? Does it usually begin as a result of pressure being put on the area? Does it come about as a result of awkward positioning? Does the pain increase or decrease with sexual excitement?
- How much pain is involved and what is it like? Is it a burning pain, a deep aching pain, or does some other description fit better? Is there anything that lessens the pain during lovemaking?
- Does the pain have specific physiological sexual effects on the one who experiences it? For example, does it lead to difficulty in maintaining an erection? Vaginal dryness? Tenseness that prevents sexual pleasure? Something else?

By clarifying what you or your partner with pain is feeling and how it is affecting your lovemaking, the two of you will be better equipped to understand how to effectively manage the pain while also increasing pleasure.

---

Cupid's Point

What are some questions that you and your partner could ask yourselves to help you understand chronic pain's effects beyond just the physiological so to include other dimensions of your relationship?

A couple of suggestions:

- How is your *communication* in bed (relational dimension) affected by the presence of pain?
- How is each of your *attitudes* (psychological dimension) toward sexuality affected by the pain?
- How is your ability to pleasure (sensual dimension) each other affected by the presence of pain?

What other relevant questions can you think of?

---

This understanding will also help in talking to your doctor. I strongly advise you, or your partner if he or she is the one who experiences the pain, consult with your physician about the ways in which chronic pain impinges on your sex life. To help make those consultations productive, you must be able to tell your doctor the particulars of the pain and its physiological effects.

A second reason it can be difficult for partners to identify just how recurrent pain is affecting their sex life is that there are many different ways in which pain can adversely affect sexual pleasure. In chapter two we learned that chronic pain relates to sexual satisfaction in four dimensions: the physiological, psychological, relational, and sensual. The physiological effects of pain are usually fairly evident and can be communicated with a little effort. But how pain affects a couple's sex life in the other three dimensions may be less transparent. Remember Howard and Barbara? They had little comprehension about the ways in which Howard's chronic pain and subsequent behavior were affecting them psychologically, relationally, or sensually.

Maybe you and your partner though are different in this respect. Perhaps the way pain impinges on your sexual relationship is simple and straightforward. But don't make that assumption unless you're sure. It's wise to begin with the idea that Cupid's Challenge may be arising for you in some ways that are more hidden. You may need to do a thorough examination of how pain detracts from your sex life in order to understand what those ways are.

Each chapter focuses on one or more kinds of problem, such as poor communication, too much anxiety during sex, or lack of sensual savvy. As you read each chapter, pay close attention to whether the problems and issues it refers to are present in your own situation. Share your thoughts with your partner and get his or her feedback.

Fulfilling the first step of *ICE* may take a concerted effort. As you clarify what the problems are, you may find them to be relatively simple. Perhaps only a few small changes can get your love life back on track. On the other hand, you may discover that the difficulties are more widespread and complex than you had realized. If so, don't get discouraged. Don't throw up your hands in an attitude of helpless-ness. This is the time for you to commit yourselves to learning effec-tive ideas that can rejuvenate your love life.

## The Second Stage of *ICE—Choose*
Once you and your partner have a clear idea about the ways in which Cupid's Challenge is impinging on your sex life, it's time for the next step of *ICE—Choose.* This is where you two discuss how best to address the problems you identified in the first step, and then begin choosing effective strategies for dealing with those problem. The *Choose* stage of *ICE* requires two basic activities:

- First, become familiar with a range of ideas for coping with how chronic pain is affecting your sexual happiness.
- Second, openly discuss the various ideas and strategies with your partner and then decide which ones seem to best fit your situation. For many couples, talking with each other about such matters can be difficult. Due to taboos and embarrassment, you and your partner may find it hard to broach the two central issues of Cupid's Challenge—pain and sexual dysfunction. As a result, you may feel inhibited when it comes to discussing which strategies might enable the two of you to improve your sex life despite chronic pain.

Since communication between partners is usually something that can be improved upon, I suggest you both skip ahead now and read chapter seven, The Arrow of Communication, before continuing on to the other chapters. There, you will find strategies to make it easier to talk about some ideas. In particular, you will learn about the concept of Clear, Caring Communication, which can guide your discussions and make them more productive.

One of the greatest benefits of the *Choose* step of *ICE* is that when partners start talking to one another about how to build a happier sex life, the discussion itself is likely to bring them closer. And when it comes to scintillating sex, closer is better! Again, recall Howard and

Barbara. One of their most serious problems was poor communication. Not only did this prevent them from understanding their situation and doing something about it, their silence was a chasm that separated them from one another. When partners come together to talk about renewing their sex life while also coping with chronic pain, they are bridging that chasm of silence. By joining together to work on an issue that is important to both of them, they are doing something that already promotes a more satisfying sexual relationship.

---

Cupid's Point

Communication is part of all three stages of *ICE,* which suggests that good communication is very important in effectively addressing Cupid's Challenge.

Does communication receive this amount of emphasis in your relationship? Do you feel that for you and your partner good communication is a key to addressing how chronic pain affects your sex life? Why or why not?

---

### The Third Step of *ICE—Explore*

You've identified the problem(s). You, and your partner too, hopefully, have skipped ahead and read chapter seven on communications and discovered some promising strategies for addressing the problem(s). And the two of you have spent quality time discussing those strategies and choosing which ones seem best for your situation. So far, however, it's been all talk. Necessary talk, yes. But only talk. Now it's time to start putting that talk into action. And that brings us to the all-important third step of *ICE, Explore.*

The *Explore* step is just what the name suggests. It's where you and your partner try out ideas that you chose in step two. Some of the strategies may be sensual ones. For these, the natural place to do your explorations is usually in the bedroom.

This kind of sensual exploration is often delightful. It can help refresh your sex life and bring back excitement that you two may have lost. However, for some partners it can also be unnerving. People tend to fall into patterns of behavior in which they do the same things in the same way, sometimes for decades. This is also true of sexual behaviors. Many couples develop a certain pattern of having sex early in their relationship and keep repeating that pattern for years. As a result, trying new activities in the bedroom can cause one or both partners to feel embarrassed, self-conscious, or anxious.

It doesn't have to be that way. Exploring new activities that may alleviate pain and increase sensuality need not be psychologically stressful if lovers go about it in the right way. They can avoid much potential anxiety and self-consciousness by agreeing to follow certain principles in their explorations. Talking about and coming to agreement on those rules can be an important part of the *Explore* step of *ICE*. Here are several guidelines that can help lubricate the wheels of sensual exploration:

- Make sure that you both understand and agree with what you are going to do and how the explorations will proceed. You want this to be a joint undertaking, not one in which one partner decides unilaterally what the other is "supposed" to like.
- Talk to each other about any doubts that either partner may have concerning the proposed activities. Be honest and support one another emotionally.
- Create a relaxing, sensual, and light mood as you explore various possibilities. Sexual pleasure thrives best in an atmosphere that is relaxed, nonjudgmental, and lighthearted.

Be patient with yourself and your partner as you try new things. The purpose of the *Explore* step is to discover which activities can create greater sexual satisfaction for both of you, so impatience won't help you fulfill that plan. An outbreak of annoyance from either partner can destroy a sexy mood very quickly. And that's true whether you direct your impatience toward yourself or your partner.

Make communication with your partner an ongoing part of the *Explore* step. The purpose of sensual exploration is to discover whether new activities can help reduce pain and increase sexual pleasure, and the only way to find out whether that's happening is to communicate with each other. This can be done in different ways. You and your lover may decide to talk afterward about how much you enjoyed a particular experience. Or, you may provide each other with continuous feedback on what you like as the activities unfold. This kind of ongoing communication—which may include sighs, soft words, and bodily movements that indicate what feels good—can be another highly sensual aspect of your encounter.

It's important for the partner who is living with pain to check with his or her physician about the suitability of any proposed new sensual activities. Your doctor can be your pain management partner and an invaluable resource as you deal with the effects of chronic pain on your sex life. Make sure to ask for and follow his or her advice about which positions, activities, and innovations are suitable given your condition.

So far we've talked about exploring sensuality in the bedroom. However, the *Explore* stage of *ICE* can also be applied outside the bedroom to deal with Cupid's Challenge as it presents itself in other dimensions. You and your partner might decide, for example, to explore new ways of relating in your everyday lives outside of the bedroom in order to increase your sense of togetherness. Or you might choose to explore overall health strategies to reduce pain levels or increase the energy available for sexual activities.

For such nonsensual explorations, too, ongoing communication is crucial. Continue talking about what you are doing in your lives that is new, how you are doing it, and what difference it is making in your love life. You will likely find that some of your explorations, sensual or otherwise, will be right on the mark.

## After *ICE,* More *ICE*

What comes after *ICE*? The answer is more *ICE.* Except the letters now stand for three new, related ideas: *Integrate, Consolidate,* and *Explore Some More.*

By *Integrate,* I simply mean to put the knowledge you gain about which strategies work best for you into a single unified framework. That framework is the four-dimensional view that you learned about in chapter two. Ideally, this will result in an integrated and effective set of strategies.

*Consolidate* means to continually improve on the strategies that you develop. Keep communicating about how to make them speak to your lives. For example, if you find that certain health strategies decrease pain and increase pleasure in your sexual activities, then build on that knowledge. Look for similar strategies that can help you make even more progress and keep communicating about the ideas that work. Help each other to stay enthusiastic and committed to an intimate bond.

By *Explore Some More,* I mean just that. Keep looking for and talking about valuable new ideas to decrease pain and increase pleasure in the bedroom. When you find something that looks promising, try it out—with your physician's approval, of course. This can help keep your sex life fresh and provide an even larger repertoire of activities to increase sensuality and intimacy while managing pain.

Continuing to explore is also something you will hopefully do outside the bedroom. There is no perfectly harmonious relationship. There are always avenues through which partners can increase their communication, closeness, and enjoyment of each other in their everyday lives. Improvements in these areas are often positively reflected in the bedroom as well. So keep at it on all fronts! Remember, when you are working together to become closer, that in itself helps to strengthen your bond.

## A Quick Review of *ICE*

Here, briefly, is the essence of the *ICE* method:

*Identify.* Identify the ways in which chronic pain is impinging on your sexual relationship. Be specific. Try to understand how pain is affecting you and your partner in all four dimensions—physiological, psychological, relational, and sensual. Then commit yourselves to addressing the problems in each dimension.

*Choose.* Talk with your partner about various strategies for dealing with Cupid's Challenge as it presents itself in your relationship. Which strategies seem most promising for each dimension? Choose strategies that best fit your situation.

*Explore.* Explore your strategies. In the bedroom, explore sensual ideas for reducing pain and increasing pleasure. Make sure that you and your partner agree to follow sound principles to make your explorations as stress-free and enjoyable as possible. Consult with your physician and follow his or her advice before undertaking any new positions or activities that may aggravate a painful condition or be physiologically stressful.

Both inside and outside the bedroom, explore strategies for dealing with Cupid's Challenge as it affects your relationship in other dimensions. Look for ways to increase your communication and your enjoyment of your lives together. Improvements in these areas can go a long way to enhancing your sex life.

## Then Continue *ICE*

- *Integrate* the strategies that work for you into a unified set of activities for addressing Cupid's Challenge in its various dimensions.
- *Consolidate* by strengthening and expanding the ideas that work best for you and your partner.

- *Explore Some More* by talking about and exploring new promising strategies both in and out of the bedroom.

Those are the basics of the *ICE* method. All that's needed now is information and ideas that will allow you and your partner to enact the method. And that's what the next nine chapters are for.

So let's get started! Let's learn about Cupid's many powerful arrows and how to sharpen them. And remember: to make more satisfying sex a reality, it's important to always keep a little *ICE* close by!

# Chapter Four

# The Arrow of Health

We are about to embark on an important journey. Our objective is to develop a multidimensional approach to Cupid's Challenge that you and your partner can tailor to your own situation. Our ultimate destination, of course, is a happier, more pleasurable, and more fully satisfying sexual experience in the face of chronic pain.

But where to begin? Are any of the four dimensions that we learned about earlier—the physiological, psychological, relational, and sensual—more fundamental than the others?

Yes. At the most basic level, pain and sexual pleasure are physiological phenomena. Though each is closely related to the other three dimensions too, they are, first and foremost, matters of the body. It stands to reason then that we should begin our journey by exploring the physiological dimension of Cupid's Challenge. Accordingly, in this chapter we will learn strategies for creating a bodily environment that can (1) help you manage your chronic pain, and (2) enhance your libido, sexual performance, and sexual pleasure.

In particular, we will focus on your physical health, especially the health of the partner who is actually living with chronic pain. However, most of the ideas here are meant for both partners. That's because good health is a value that should encompass your entire relationship. Strategies to achieve a healthy lifestyle are among Cupid's most fundamental tools for creating a scintillating sex life regardless of chronic pain. Together, they form one of your and your partner's most potent weapons—The Arrow of Health.

## The Physiology of Pain and of Pleasure

To comprehend the important role that good health plays in addressing Cupid's Challenge, it will help to understand some of the basics of both pain and pleasure. Let's begin by focusing for a moment on the nature of pain.

Pain comes in different forms, but in each case, it originates from external or internal stimuli that affect nerve endings. In most circumstances pain is an indication of injury or undue stress to some part of the body. But sometimes pain signals continue to be generated even after the injured part has healed or the stress has been alleviated.

To comprehend this difference, it helps to consider an example. If you inadvertently touch a hot plate with your fingers, you react immediately by withdrawing your hand. At the same time, pain signals travel via your nerves from the spot of the injury up through your spinal cord until they reach a part of your brain named the *thalamus.* There, the signals are translated into a conscious experience of pain. That experience can vary widely depending on the injury or bodily disturbance that is involved. In the case of touching a hot plate, the pain typically takes the form of a sharp burning sensation that becomes less intense after a few seconds. In other cases, the pain may likely be described in another way. There are several main parameters that are useful for describing the experience of pain:

- Quality. This consists of two parts: (1) the nature of the pain sensation, for example whether it's piercing, dull, throbbing, or achy; and (2) the intensity of the pain.
- Duration. How long the pain continues without letting up.
- Frequency. How often the pain recurs, for example every day, every hour, or every few minutes.
- Exacerbations. Factors that initiate the pain or make it worse.
- Alleviations. Factors that lessen the pain or make it go away.

In many cases, the experience of pain includes a clear indication of the pain generator—the bodily location of the pain. Sometimes, however, it can be difficult to pinpoint the pain's exact location.

The uncomfortable experience caused by touching a hot plate is called *acute* pain. Generally, for such pain the brain quickly begins generating signals that inhibit the painful sensation. This negative feedback loop is a natural protective mechanism that our body employs to reduce and eventually stop the pain. In some cases, however, the loop doesn't work well. For instance, when chemical receptors inhibit the stop mechanism and the brain continues to perceive the pain signals as before. At the same time, chemicals may be released that cause inflammation and even more pain; and this may result over time in chronic pain. Chemicals that affect other places in the body are also often released when the pain occurs, including ones that cause feelings of stress, anxiety, and even depression.

Sexuality, too, is based on physiology. Central aspects of sexuality such as libido (sexual desire) and capacity for sexual gratification are greatly affected by chemicals called hormones, especially testosterone and progesterone. These sex hormones start becoming prominent at puberty and are strongly active during the late teens, twenties, and thirties. Typically, hormone activity gradually decreases with age. Still, even with lower hormone levels, many older couples continue to enjoy an active and satisfying sex life.

The sensual pleasures that attend sexuality are physiologically-based. For almost all women and men there are certain areas of the body that are sensitive and respondent to appropriate touch, kissing, and manipulation. For women, these erogenous zones typically include lips, breasts, nipples, the vulvar area, and the clitoris. For men, they most often include the penis and testicles. For both women and men, there may also be other areas of the body that are erotically sensitive.

Erogenous zones tend to be highly vascularized, which is to say they encompass numerous blood vessels. As a result, when the individual, whether man or woman is sexually excited, these areas become engorged with blood. Sexual excitement may also cause lubricating fluid to be secreted as nature's way of preparing the man and woman for intercourse.

## The Value of Overall Health for Pain Management and Sexual Pleasure

Because pain on the one hand and sexual desire and pleasure on the other are both bodily phenomena, each of these kinds of experiences can be strongly influenced by your overall health. An obvious example of how good health can affect pain levels and the duration of pain is the ability of a well-functioning immune system to speed the healing of an injury. This, in turn, can result in less pain being associated with the injury over time. An example of how good health conduces to good sex is improved blood flow having a dramatic bearing on a man's ability to maintain an erection. Likewise, improved blood flow for his mate can increase the sensitivity of her erogenous zones and lead to greater sensual pleasure.

These examples are only the tip of a large and vitally important iceberg—or perhaps I should say, *heatberg*—that you and your partner could benefit from being aware of. If chronic pain is making a serious nuisance of itself in your bedroom and sexual pleasure is being shortchanged, health-related strategies can be one of your most effective means for improving the situation.

Unfortunately, modern culture presents many roadblocks that violate sound health principles in everyday living. As a consequence, making good health a priority may require some lifestyle changes. Fortunately, that's often not as difficult as it may seem. Making such changes is typically a matter of breaking old, counterproductive habits and replacing them with new, health-efficacious ones. That may take a little patience, but the results are well worth the wait.

For a broad range of habits, a general rule of thumb is that it takes twenty-one days to break one. It is reassuring to know that your commitment to walking down a new road for three weeks can lead to permanent lifestyle changes to strongly enhance the quality of your life, not to mention increase your life span as well. The rewards of improved health—including greater energy, less pain, and increased feelings of wellbeing and self-efficacy—far outweigh the perceived inconveniences. For those dealing with chronic pain in the bedroom, making the change to a healthier lifestyle is the epitome of a "no-brainer."

Below are highlighted some of the most important elements of a healthy lifestyle. For each of these, you will learn how healthy practices can make a very positive difference as you deal with Cupid's Challenge. You will also find ideas for how you and your partner can maximize each of these elements in your lives.

## Eat for Health, Pain Management, and Sexier Sex

Good health is a matter of balance. A system out of balance is a system that is more vulnerable to injury and illness; it is also less able to heal quickly and more susceptible to pain and continuing pain. It's one in which bodily resources that could be used for pleasurable sexual activity are less available as well.

Balance begins with the food and drink we take into our bodily system. What we put into our mouths at the breakfast bar, the luncheonette, and the dinner table can make an enormous difference in energy, stamina, capacity to fight off disease, and ability to manage pain. Ironically, some people who appear to be extremely well fed are actually starving various parts of their bodies by eating an imbalanced diet.

There are two main ways our unhealthy dietary habits can contribute to us losing our balance. The first occurs when we consistently consume the wrong number of calories. The second happens when we consume calories in the wrong forms and proportions. Let's take each kind of bodily "imbalancing acts" in turn.

### Too Little or Too Much

A crucial part of maintaining dietary balance is to take in the right number of calories in relation to your needs for energy and bodily maintenance. When there is an imbalance in this respect, it sometimes takes the form of too few calories consumed. When this occurs consistently over time, you may lose so much weight that your bodily resources and energy-generating capabilities are depleted. This can result in less capacity for fighting off pain-producing illness as well as promoting healing.

Starving the body also negatively affects libido and sexual pleasure. Sexual activity requires both physical and mental energy, but when the body is constantly hungry, there may be little energy available for sex. The meager calories available are allocated to functions that are immediately important, such as bodily maintenance and staying mentally alert. As a result, there is a decreased enthusiasm for sex and less enjoyment when it occurs.

Caloric imbalance more frequently occurs in the other direction, with the individual regularly ingesting more calories than are needed. These excess calories are stored as fat, and eventually obesity results. This is a common threat for individuals who are dealing with chronic pain. Over and over I see patients who use food to try to deaden or alleviate their pain. In actuality, their overeating often does just the opposite by aggravating the condition that gives rise to their discomfort.

This is most obvious in situations where pain originates from joints or other structural elements of the body due to conditions such as arthritis or lower back complications. In such cases, added pounds typically mean added stress on the weakened parts of the body, which may then exacerbate the pain. Carrying around excess weight can also worsen and extend pain for other ailments too. Even headache pain can be intensified and lengthened due to symptoms of obesity such as fatigue and high blood pressure.

In the bedroom, being overweight tends to have a number of repercussions that are detrimental to individuals who are dealing with chronic pain:

- Carrying around unneeded pounds takes extra energy, thus less energy becomes available for sex.
- Being overweight often contributes to a more sedentary lifestyle, which also decreases the energy and stamina available for sexual activity.

- Blood circulation can be negatively affected by excess fat. This can lead to inhibited blood flow in the erogenous zones, which may in turn result in reduced sexual readiness, performance, and pleasure.
- Added weight means added pressure on various parts of the body. This can cause pain to erupt more often and more seriously in bed, especially if the condition causing the pain is structurally related.
- Flexibility and ability to enjoy various positions while having sex typically suffer with obesity. These limitations can be particularly troublesome if the ability to move freely is also compromised by the condition causing the pain.

In sum, it's clear that carrying too little or too much weight in relation to bodily needs can present a major obstacle to achieving better sex with less pain. If weight issues are a factor in your bedroom, an excellent place to begin dealing with them is at your physician's office. Your doctor can advise you (or your partner if he or she has a weight problem) on your optimum weight and help you determine an appropriate diet to get your intake of calories more in line with your output.

This may seem like obvious advice, but often what's most obvious is also most important. Please don't overlook weight control as a vitally important weapon for dealing with Cupid's Challenge. Keeping weight within healthy parameters is one of the most potentially effective tools for improving health, managing chronic pain, and enhancing sexual pleasure.

### The Well-fueled Machine

The second area where your diet can create a bodily imbalance is closely related to the first, and it's probably even more common than taking in too few or too many calories. This is the problem of eating the wrong kinds of food or in the wrong proportions. It's one thing to consume the correct number of calories. It's another to make sure they are the right kinds of calories.

Achieving the proper balance of proteins, carbohydrates, and fats for energy and proper bodily functioning is something many of us learned about in school. But while the lessons are often ignored in the course of daily living, they never go out of date. Consider this analogy: We all know that a machine such as a car has to be correctly fueled and oiled in order to function properly. When the wrong kind of gas or oil is used, various parts of the machine lose efficiency and may even break down. And because all elements of the machine are interconnected, when one part runs into trouble, others are affected.

The same basic ideas apply to you and me. If we consistently put the wrong fuel (the wrong mixture of proteins, carbohydrates, and fats) into the wonderful machine that is our body, we can expect trouble spots to eventually arise. The trouble might be in the form of high cholesterol causing arterial plaque, elevated blood pressure, or reduced immune system effectiveness. Whatever the problems, they will likely have repercussions through much of the rest of the system.

Another excellent example of how millions of people make poor eating choices day after day is the high per capita rate of sugar consumption in the United States. Sugar overconsumption can cause serious problems with our metabolism, which is a kind of slow fire that burns constantly throughout our body turning food into heat and other forms of energy. Consuming too much sugar is like throwing gasoline into the metabolic fire. The fire flares up because our body metabolizes the sugar too fast and our normal metabolic processes turn into a kind of wildfire. This wildfire includes sparks that consist of free radicals created by the metabolism of sugar. When these free radicals enter our cells, they can weaken protective mechanisms and cause the DNA transcription process that occurs during cell division to misfire, which can in turn lead to serious diseases such as hypertension and cancer.

---

**Cupid's Point**

Many who live with chronic pain find that certain dietary elements such as processed sugar, caffeine, or overly fatty meals have an adverse effect on their pain levels and the duration of painful episodes. How balanced is your diet? If you are living with chronic pain, have you ever found that what you eat makes the discomfort worsen? Or that it reduces the pain?

How about sexual activity? Do you ever find that your desire for sex or the energy you have available for sex is affected by what you eat? If so, which foods and what are their effects?

---

For those of us who must deal with chronic pain, the consequences of an imbalanced diet can be especially troublesome. What weakens the system as a whole also tends to adversely affect whatever condition is leading to pain. It may even cause the pain to increase in severity and length, and to become more resistant to medications and other methods of relief. The condition will have its best chance of improving if we take steps to restore balance by making the surrounding bodily environment as healthy as possible. Again, this means the entire machine must be properly fueled.

A proper diet is also crucial for the most enjoyable sex. Many bodily elements come into play during exciting and pleasurable sexual experiences. You can think of the purely physiological part of sex as being like a chain in which hormones, blood vessels, skin, neurotransmitters, muscles, and other bodily features all play their important roles. Each element requires its proper nutrients in order to work optimally. And, as the old saying goes, a chain is truly only as strong as its weakest link. If some link in the chain is not getting the nutrients it needs to do its job, it will become starved. And that starvation will tend to disrupt the chain of events that underlie the sexual experience.

To strengthen the chain you must ensure that all of the bodily elements that make for good sex are getting their proper nutrients through a well-balanced diet. Don't take it for granted that you are getting the nutrition you need each day. In order to maximize your chances for success in eating well, it's important to create a well-designed plan.

An excellent way to start designing a diet that optimally meets your nutritional requirements is to talk to your doctor or other health professional. When you do, ask about the general dietary guidelines below. You've probably heard of some of these before. But there's a reason why these rules are repeated again and again: they work!

- Make it a practice to eat a wide variety of fresh fruits and vegetables.
- Minimize your intake of processed sugars.
- Opt for whole grains instead of processed grains.
- Choose complex over simple carbohydrates.
- Go nutty! Many nuts are excellent sources of the healthiest fats.
- Choose lean over fatty meats.
- Minimize your intake of saturated fats; foods and oils that contain fat of the unsaturated variety are a healthier choice.
- Go easy on salt; make it a practice to read labels to determine the sodium content of foods.
- Be judicious in your caffeine consumption; choose decaffeinated beverages when you can.

For a set of further dietary guidelines that I call "Making a Better Choice" and often give to my patients, please see Appendix A.

## The Power of Exercise

Another essential element in achieving physiological balance is exercise. Combined with proper diet, exercise can be one of your most valuable tools for addressing Cupid's Challenge.

We can again use the analogy of the body as a machine to understand the critical role exercise plays in good health. Machines are built to fulfill some purpose. Of course there's nothing wrong with a machine, say an automobile or a jet, being aesthetically pleasing in design too. But automobiles are meant to be driven, and jets to fly, and if the machine just sits in the garage or the hangar looking pretty, it's not fulfilling its proper function or realizing its full potential.

Much the same goes for the exquisite machine that is your body. All human bodies are meant to be physically active to keep their muscles strong and toned, whether that comes from exercise or recreational activities. If we are seldom active, if we just sit in a "garage" consisting of an easy chair or couch while exerting as little physical effort as possible, we will quickly start doing the human equivalent of rusting. Our muscles, including our heart, will begin to weaken, our circulation will become sluggish, our skin will lose tone, and our internal organs will lose efficiency. In short, our entire body will begin deteriorating. The adage "Use it or lose it!" definitely applies here.

Not only does the body gradually deteriorate without appropriate exercise, its various components—such as the hormonal, neurological, and circulatory systems—tend to get out of balance within themselves and with each other. This often spells trouble for the chronic pain survivor because it may exacerbate their condition leading to the pain. Plus, healing can become more difficult, recovery harder, and the pain more persistent.

Sufficient exercise also promotes healthy sexual functioning. System imbalances caused by a lack of exercise can seriously disrupt the chain of physiological events that lead to sexual pleasure and satisfaction. Conversely, by getting adequate exercise you help to strengthen the chain in many areas including reducing cholesterol, improving circulation, stimulating hormone production, increasing stamina, and producing a heightened sense of wellbeing.

Given all of this, it's clear that exercise is as important as diet for keeping your body in balance and for addressing Cupid's Challenge effectively. Really, the question isn't whether or not to exercise, but rather what kind and how frequently.

Are you and your partner doing well on the exercise front? If you work, then unless you're a professional athlete, chances are your job is relatively physically undemanding, or your duties require the exercise of only a few parts of your body such as your legs if you are standing a lot. In addition, the physical demands of maintaining a home are often less now than they were in the past. Though most of us are thankful for clothes dryers, dishwashers, powerful vacuum systems, and no-iron clothes, these conveniences have the downside of contributing to a more sedentary lifestyle.

Our leisure time activities also often present few physical challenges. Reading, watching television or movies, surfing the internet, and chatting with our friends on the phone may or may not be mentally edifying. But such activities can leave our bodies gasping for a physical challenge.

The problem of getting enough exercise in a normal day can be especially serious for those living with chronic pain. For one thing, whatever condition is leading to the pain may limit the individual's mobility and make some forms of exercise difficult or impossible. Also, the experience of pain or the fear that energetic activity will lead to greater discomfort may make exercise seem unattractive. That's why it's important to understand that for almost all individuals and situations there are effective exercises that are doable and relatively pain-free.

As with diet, the best place to begin designing an exercise plan that's appropriate for you or your partner is your physician's office. As you talk to your doctor, be aware that there are three basic kinds of exercise: aerobic, anaerobic, and skill building:

- Aerobic exercise is bodily movement that conditions your heart and lungs by increasing your body's efficiency at using oxygen. It includes such activities as walking, jogging, bicycling, and swimming.

- Anaerobic exercise is for maintaining and increasing muscle mass. It typically involves short sessions of very demanding activity such as lifting weights and sprint swimming.
- Skill building exercise helps to improve coordination, balance, and muscle tone. Such exercises include yoga, golf, and tai chi.

All three varieties are important for good health, though aerobic exercise is probably the most crucial because of its vitalness to the heart, lungs, and circulation. However, the particular kinds of exercise that are most appropriate, as well as the proper intensity of the exercise, will vary greatly among individuals. For example, many weight-bearing exercises may be inappropriate for individuals with back or joint problems. Ask your doctor to advise you about which forms of exercise are most important for you and to suggest specific activities that are suitable for your condition and current fitness level. You may also benefit from speaking with a physical therapist, a knowledgeable certified fitness trainer, or an athletic trainer. Note that many physical activities involve two or even all three kinds of exercise.

Some individuals prefer an exercise program that makes use of dedicated apparatus such as a stationary bicycle or treadmill, which can be adjusted to match your fitness level. Other people find that they are able to get all or a good deal of their exercise in by engaging in everyday activities such as mowing the lawn, gardening, rearranging the living room, or biking the few miles to and from work. Still others find that a mixture of everyday activities with more structured exercises such as dance aerobics or yoga works best for them.

Here are some guidelines and other ideas that can be useful as you develop an exercise program that fits your needs and lifestyle:

Start gently. Don't bite off too much at first. Pay attention to what your body is telling you and build up gradually over time. For exercises such as free walking, treadmill walking, and bicycling, I often suggest to my patients that they begin with three sets per day, with each set lasting two to seven minutes. They may then gradually increase this until they can do twenty to thirty minutes at a time, for a total of thirty to forty-five minutes per day. Here again, talk to your physician about how specifically to pace yourself in your program.

Choose activities that you enjoy. If you find riding a stationary bicycle or walking on a treadmill to be tedious, you might consider swimming, biking, or jogging as alternatives that offer greater variety and stimulation. Or, if doing simple stretching exercises seems monotonous, you may find that immersing yourself in the mental and physical discipline of yoga or pilates keeps your interest piqued. Designing a personal exercise program that's fun and interesting makes sense because the more enjoyable it is, the more likely you will stick with it.

Exercise on a frequent and regular schedule. Instead of undertaking a brief period of activity a couple of times a month, try to make exercise a frequent and steady part of your life. Exercising moderately three, four, or more times a week on a set schedule will likely provide more benefit than engaging in more intensive exercise that is done irregularly.

Join with others. Exercise is often more enjoyable when done with a friend or in a group setting. The mutual encouragement, camaraderie, and shared sense of accomplishment that comes from being with others can make your program more fun and help you stay on track. Being with friends or a group can also enhance the psychological benefits to be gained from exercise.

Find ways to exercise with your mate. This can be an especially rewarding way to make exercise enhance your partnership. You might join a fitness group or club together. Or your joint exercise program could include everyday activities that you do with one another. Something as simple as going for a brisk half-hour walk together several evenings a week can bring substantial fitness benefits. Exercising together also tends to draw partners closer, which of course is just what Cupid is longing for! Take care, however, that whatever exercises you do jointly are appropriate for both of you.

On this same note, please remember that for couples dealing with chronic pain, exercise isn't just for the partner who is actually experiencing the pain. Ideally, both partners will get sufficient exercise, whether together or separately. The benefits of exercise—for health, increased stamina, and sexual fitness—are for both partners to enjoy.

---

Cupid's Point

Do you get sufficient exercise in your normal day? If not, consider what possibilities are available to you at your workplace. These might include walking or biking to and from work or going for a walk during your lunch hour. And how about at home? Consider what natural opportunities are present there such as walking, climbing stairs, or working in the yard. How could you and your partner change the way you typically spend your weekends in order to get more exercise?

---

Even if one partner is restricted to a wheelchair or scooter, there can be both physical and psychological benefits to couples making time to have regular outings together. This was illustrated by John, an arthritic patient of mine, who usually got around in a scooter. Still, he went out most fair-weather days on a mile-long outing through a nearby park, with his wife Lucy walking beside him. The two usually stopped once or twice during these journeys while John exercised his arms and shoulders with light weights and Lucy practiced Tai Chi. John said that he consistently found his "scooter walks" to be invigorating. He remarked that they were one of the most enjoyable parts of the day for both him and Lucy, and they had brought them closer.

## Sweet, Empowering Sleep

A third main key to approaching Cupid's Challenge with greater physiological power is to get a good night's sleep, and to do so consistently. Sleep is one of the body's most vital healing and rejuvenating mechanisms. During sleep, bodily activities are reduced to a minimum, allowing cells to repair themselves after the wear and tear that each day brings. When our sleep is insufficient, we awaken with the necessary overnight cell repairs incomplete. As a result, we feel tired and listless throughout the day. Then, because the body is not well-rested, conditions leading to pain are more susceptible to aggravation, and the pain itself seems more painful.

Chronic lack of sleep also impinges on a number of elements important for proper sexual functioning. These effects may include decreased libido, lowered hormone levels, and erectile difficulties for men. Overall, the energy and stamina that could help power a pleasurable sexual experience are compromised when we don't get enough sleep. When the body is fatigued, interest in sexual activity as well as interest in many other activities typically decreases. And why shouldn't it? Our body knows when it needs to rest, and it knows that exerting itself sexually will only increase that need.

To ensure adequate rest, maintain a regular sleep schedule. Your body is on a twenty-four-hour clock set by the sun, and regular patterns of sleep and wakefulness help to determine bodily rhythms. These are rhythms, such as hormone levels and metabolic rates, that rise and fall at regular intervals. For most people, seven to nine hours of uninterrupted sleep a night is about the right amount. Also, some people are night owls, some are morning larks. Here, as elsewhere, your body can tell you a lot if you listen to it. If you consistently wake up tired, you may not be getting enough sleep. Other indicators include a tendency to fall asleep easily during the day, near-constant drowsiness, and difficulty in concentrating.

There are a number of sleep disorders. Aside from chronic lack of sleep, the most common of these is probably sleep apnea. This typically results in snoring that may disturb the sleep not only of the individual but also of his or her partner. Sleep apnea is often associated with overeating, smoking, and other habits that are marks of poor lifestyle choices.

If you or your partner often have difficulty getting enough sleep, it's important to seek your physician's advice. First, try to identify as clearly as possible just what the problem is. For example, do you have difficulty sleeping soundly whether it's day or night? Or is it only at night when the trouble arises, leaving you to catch catnaps throughout the day? Also try to identify as clearly as possible what it is that seems to be causing the problem. By asking and answering the following questions, you may be able to determine one or more contributing factors and develop strategies to overcome them:

- Does what you eat or drink in the hours just before bed—for example, coffee, tea, chocolate, or a heavy meal—have a role in keeping you awake? Caffeine, a heavy meal, and alcohol can all cause sleep difficulties. Also, consuming beverages of any kind just before bed can lead to waking up in order to go the bathroom.
- How does your bed feel to you? Are the mattress and pillows comfortable or do they seem to aggravate the sleep problem? Do you wake up with your back or neck aching or feeling tired?
- Does your partner's behavior in bed—for example snoring, watching television, or reading with the light on—keep you awake?
- Are external sounds or sights keeping you awake or waking you from your sleep? Are the noisy neighbors in the apartment above, sirens, the television in the next room, or the glare of the streetlight outside your window interrupting your sleep?
- Is your schedule working against your natural circadian rhythms? For example, does your body seem to be telling you that you are a "night person" who has a natural tendency to stay up late and wake late, whereas your job requires you to get up early?
- Are you going to bed at such irregular times that your body has no chance to adjust to a single pattern?
- Are you catnapping so much during the day that you find it difficult to sleep at night, which in turn leads to more catnapping the next day?

- Is the temperature in your bedroom so cold or warm that you often awaken feeling chilly or too hot?

If you can identify the specific problem, then making a change or two may help power you to a more consistently restful sleep. The change could be as simple as taking the television out of the bedroom, using an eye mask, or committing yourself to going to bed at the same time every night.

Here's a second list of questions to ask about your sleep difficulties. If the answer is "yes" to any of these, be sure to seek your physician's advice:

- Is pain keeping you awake?
- Do any drugs you are taking seem to be contributing to the problem? Various drugs for a number of conditions ranging from high blood pressure to colds can make sleep more difficult.
- Are breathing problems such as snoring or irregular breathing disturbing your sleep?
- Do you lie in bed for hours, your mind going "a mile a minute"? Is the stress of daily life keeping your thoughts so riled up that insomnia results?
- Do you often have tingling sensations in your legs that make you keep wanting to move them (restless legs syndrome)?
- Is your sleep being disturbed by you having to rise several times a night to urinate? (enlarged prostate, urinary tract infection, urinary incontinence, etc.)
- Is menopause contributing to the problem? Many women who have never had sleep difficulties suddenly find insomnia to be their pillow mate when menopause arrives.

When you visit your health professional, explain the specific problem and what seems to be contributing to it as clearly as possible. This will help your doctor understand whether a condition such as sleep apnea, menopause, or stress may be at the root of the difficulty so that she can determine proper treatment. In the event that she prescribes a sleep-inducing pharmaceutical, you should be aware that some of these drugs can interfere with libido and sexual response. So be sure to ask about possible side effects that might work against you and your partner's sex life. Ask whether there are natural alternatives to these pharmaceuticals that might go a significant way toward solving the problem.

---

Cupid's Point

On a scale of one to ten, how do you rate the quality of your sleep? If you said anything less than *ten,* that's reason enough to seek out ways that can improve your sleep sessions. Here's a simple four-step process for doing so:

1. Get clear on what the problem is, when it occurs, and how often it occurs.
2. Determine what factor(s) seem to be leading to the problem.
3. Look for ways to address those factors. Enlist your partner's help for ideas. Seek the advice of your physician.
4. Apply one or more ideas. Does your sleep get better? If not, start again at step 1 or 2.

Remember, getting adequate sleep is vital for effective pain management and sexual functioning, not to mention overall functioning. Make it one of your most important health goals.

---

## Other Health Strategies

No Smoking Allowed!
For partners facing Cupid's Challenge, as for everyone else, smoking is a practice that makes no sense. First, for the chronic pain survivor, the net effect of consuming tobacco whether through cigarettes, cigars, pipes, snuffs, vapes, and all of the other ways is to create a

weakened bodily environment in which whatever condition is leading to the pain has less chance to heal. In fact, smoking may make the condition worse. In particular, smokers face increased incidences of lung cancer, emphysema, and reduced lung capacity. In addition, arterial plaque, impaired circulation, gum disease, a weakened immune system, and a greatly increased risk of heart attack and other cardiovascular disease have all been shown to result from smoking. To try to effectively manage chronic pain while continuing to smoke is like trying to walk while having your shoelaces tied together.

As for sex, cigarettes are simply not sexy. Some of the images that have been created over time by companies advertising cigarettes don't accurately represent the truth. The ads don't show the yellowed teeth and stained fingers or the acrid breath that come from smoking. More importantly, smoking results in reduced sexual performance. Its harmful effect on circulation makes it more difficult for men to attain and maintain erections and for women to enjoy full vascularization of their erogenous zones. Its injurious effect on the lungs also diminishes stamina and reduces the energy available for partners to enjoy one another in bed. And Cupid finds it difficult to aim his arrows effectively if he has to do so through a smoky haze.

If you happen to be a smoker, please find a way to give it up—the sooner the better! Tobacco is undisputedly dangerous to an individual's overall health.

## Use of Nutritional Supplements

Nutritional supplements take various forms, including vitamins, minerals, and herbs. A nutritionally adequate diet should provide you with your daily requirements, which are dependent on a number of factors such as your activity and stress levels, your age, the season, and your nutrient absorption levels. If your diet is not optimal or if a special condition warrants, a vitamin-mineral supplement may be in order.

Many claims are made about the benefits of various nutritional supplements, including testimonials about pain relief and improved sexual functioning. However, not all of these statements are backed by sound scientific research. It's extremely important to be aware, for example, that some herbs can be toxic when taken in combination with one other, or when taken with other medicines or even foods. The *Physicians' Desk Reference* is a good source for sound information on herbs and other nutritional supplements. However, your best guide is a physician or other health professional with good knowledge about supplements. I strongly suggest that you consult an informed health professional about the wisdom of adding any nutritional supplements to your diet.

While we are on the subject of medical consultations, it is vital for you to choose your healthcare professionals wisely. Not all physicians have equal knowledge about all aspects of medicine. Nor are all physicians equal in their areas of expertise. For individuals who are dealing with chronic pain, as for others, it is crucial to find a doctor who is very knowledgeable about your condition as well as someone you trust.

One useful place to begin in selecting a doctor is to ask your friends and acquaintances for referrals. But don't stop there. On your first contact, ask about the doctor's qualifications and if he or she will offer a fifteen-minute complimentary visit to discuss what you are looking for in your personal care. Ask the doctor for references, and especially for patients that he or she has treated who are willing to give testimonials. Please remember that patients must give doctors their permission to share their stories. Many times the healthcare professional's website will have pictures and testimonials of patients whose lives they have positively affected.

In researching the best doctor for yourself, pay attention to how you are treated, not only by the doctor but also by the office staff. Do office personnel take the time to get to know you? Do they consistently treat you with friendliness and respect? These are all important aspects of patient care.

Remember, your health is of highest importance, so your expectations for healthcare should be high too. If it turns out that your high expectations are not being met by your physician or by the office as a whole, then perhaps you are in the wrong office. In Appendix B you will find more on what to look for in selecting a physician.

Effects of Pharmaceuticals

Some pain medications, both prescription and nonprescription, can significantly inhibit sexual desire or performance. This fact is of special importance to couples facing Cupid's Challenge, and it should be a topic for straightforward discussion with your physician.

Learn the side effects of any pain medications that you (or your partner) are taking and how they might affect your sex life. If you discover that any of them have a tendency to negatively affect libido or sexual performance, find out if your doctor can prescribe suitable replacement medications that have no or fewer such effects. Or possibly your physician can authorize a "drug holiday"—a few days in which you need not take the medications.

If not, don't take that as a reason for giving up on addressing Cupid's Challenge. Instead, redouble your efforts to develop non-pharmaceutical methods of pain management, and seek new ways to enrich your love life despite any performance-inhibiting effects of the drugs you are taking. You will find many ideas for doing so in the chapters to come.

## Scintillating Sex Knows No Age

As we age, we generally become more susceptible to conditions that give rise to pain. At the same time, age usually brings a reduction in hormone levels, a lowered libido, and some reduction in sexual performance. As a result, a greater percentage of older couples find themselves facing Cupid's Challenge. However, by establishing a healthy lifestyle through proper diet, exercise, and sleep, they can lay the groundwork for effective pain management while creating a bodily environment that helps to enhance sexual desire and performance.

It's important to remember that what counts as scintillating sex for a couple may change with time. The nature and frequency of activities that bring partners sexual pleasure and satisfaction in their sixties and seventies may be considerably different from what did the job in their twenties and thirties. A less "acrobatic" sex life, one with more holding, cuddling, and caressing, if those are the activities that bring the couple sexual happiness, can still be beautiful and life-affirming.

Mature couples are also becoming increasingly aware of pharmaceutical options that have been developed to help enhance sexual performance. One problem that plagues many of these couples is the greater difficulty a man may have in maintaining an erection as he becomes older. New erection-enhancing drugs have made great inroads into managing this problem. If you are a man of any age who is having erectile difficulties, explain your symptoms to your physician and ask whether any of the new drugs are right for you.

For women, the persistent vaginal dryness that often accompanies hormonal changes can be treated in several ways. Often, something so simple as applying water-based lubricants can make a difference. Your prescribing health professional can advise you on possible pharmaceutical options for other problems caused by hormonal changes. Note that bioidentical hormone replacement therapy (BHRT) can also be an alternative to pharmaceutical hormone replacement for some individuals.

Maintaining a healthy lifestyle should always be a prime goal for older couples. This is all the more true for couples, no matter their age, in which one or both partners are dealing with chronic pain. The more years we put behind us, the more important it is to follow basic health principles such as seeing our physician regularly, maintaining a healthy diet, and getting sufficient exercise and sleep. If you and your partner are committed to addressing Cupid's Challenge effectively, it is vital to follow through with taking action. And the proper way to begin dealing with the dimensions of Cupid's Challenge is to develop a comprehensive action plan that touches all of these main aspects of your health.

Then implementing that plan is your most important step in becoming a more effective manager for your chronic pain as well as for achieving optimal health. It is also the keystone for creating a strong foundation for achieving a happier sex life. By doing so, you will make Cupid a happy fellow!

# Chapter Five

# The Arrow of Attitude

In Cupid's wonderful quiver, there is no more powerful tool for increasing your sexual delight even when living with chronic pain than an affirmative attitude. In fact, avoiding negativity and embracing affirmation can help you and your partner make attitude your friend, not your foe, in bed. In particular, there are four crucial areas where an affirmative attitude can help you manage the impact of chronic pain on your sex life:

- Your pain.
- Sex and your sexuality.
- Yourself.
- Your partnership.

## What Is an Affirmative Attitude?

An *affirmative* attitude is one that incorporates four basic characteristics: it's realistic, hopeful, action-oriented, and empowering. Let's take a moment to go into some detail about each of these aspects so we can better understand what to aim for.

### An Affirmative Attitude Is Realistic

For some people, having an affirmative attitude means seeing everything as perpetually rosy. They think that to bring up or even to admit to some problem or issue in their lives would amount to expressing negativity. I occasionally come across individuals like this in pain-troubled relationships. These are cases in which one or both partners refuse to deal with their problem because they think that admitting to it would be a problem in itself.

But nothing could be further from the truth. Recognizing that we have a problem is not a form of negativity. On the contrary, it's the first step toward doing something about the problem. In fact, ignoring a difficulty in some misguided effort not to appear negative or not to rock the boat is an excellent way to help ensure that the problem will continue—and possibly even get worse.

That's why in developing an affirmative attitude toward Cupid's Challenge, it's important for you and your partner to make a realistic appraisal of how the challenge arises in your life. This means, as I suggested earlier in discussing the *ICE* method, evaluating the problem in terms of how it affects all four dimensions—physiological, psychological, relational, and sensual. Here we can see how taking that step is part of developing an affirmative attitude toward managing how pain affects your sex life.

## An Affirmative Attitude Dares to Dream

After acknowledging present realities, an affirmative attitude turns to the future with hope. When you and your partner take on this attitude about improving your sex life, you are looking to a brighter tomorrow and expecting to find effective ways to deal with the issues confronting you. You are daring to dream.

Not daring to dream is all too common among individuals and couples living with chronic pain. They sometimes even find advocates among their family or friends for their gloomy viewpoint. Maybe you've met the kind of "realist" who denigrates taking a hopeful stance toward the future. These are the cynics who will tell you, in regard to some matter, that things will never get better, that there's nothing anyone can do to make them so, and that if you think otherwise you're being unrealistic. Well, sorry cynics. It's you who are being unrealistic. In fact, by assuming that there is nothing you can do to improve your situation, you help ensure the status quo.

Having hope for the future is a thoroughly realistic viewpoint because hope is what empowers people to create the future. If your attitude is an engine that can help take you to happier sexual experiences, hope is its fuel. After beginning with a realistic appraisal of your circumstances, then pour hope into your engine and start searching for ways to better your situation. The idea is to keep the engine of attitude fueled up, and then keep applying what you learn until you get to where you want to be.

Unfortunately, many people get bogged down in ruminating about past difficulties or in grappling with present ones. They then allow those problems to define their self-image or their idea of what's possible. This was well-illustrated by the plight of Ron, a man in his forties who came to me beset by shoulder and neck pain that he had experienced for almost a decade. As we talked, it came out that his sexual relationship with his wife had suffered greatly due to this chronic pain. Over the past several years they had attempted to have sex only rarely because of his discomfort, until eventually they stopped trying, and had not had sex for over a year.

Ron tried to rationalize the situation. But his comments suggested that one factor in the couple's abstinence might be his having developed a negative image of himself as a sexual person. "I've learned to live with it," he said at one point. "But you know doctor, I don't really mind so much. After all, if I can't keep it up, maybe it's time to give it up." He then laughed at his self-deprecating joke.

After our talk, I prescribed a new pain medication he had not tried before. When I saw him a month later, he wowed me with stories of how well it had worked for him. But when I asked him if the pain relief had been sufficient to allow him to renew his sexual relationship with his wife, he surprised me by saying that he had not approached her, had not even talked to her about sex, since our last visit.

When I asked why, he said, "I'd like to try again, but there are so many things on my mind these days—finances, the kids' college, retirement not being where we expected it to be." After a pause he added, "And maybe I'm a little scared, too. Because I've failed so many times before."

It was evident that Ron's attitude toward himself in relation to sex was based on past negative experiences and those were preventing him from joining his wife in trying to create a more fulfilling sexual relationship once his pain was less severe. We can take an important lesson from Ron's case: in approaching Cupid's Challenge, don't allow yourself to be defined by the very problems you are confronting. Instead, define yourself as a person who is focused on solving those problems.

I've found that people with a negative attitude about dealing effectively with chronic pain, and with Cupid's Challenge in particular, also exhibit negativity toward other aspects of life. If this describes you or your partner, it's important to seek ways to cultivate a more hopeful, forward-looking attitude. There are many actions you can take and habits you can develop to help you embrace this positive outlook as you deal with Cupid's Challenge. A few examples include:

- Learn from the past, but don't brood over it. Your past should be a friend to guide your future, not an enemy to sabotage it.
- Make each night a positive transition. When you go to bed, think of what was good that day. Let go of what was not so good. Anticipate tomorrow and then sleep well to prepare for it.
- Welcome the openness of the new day. Wake each morning realizing that what's possible for you today is a joy-filled surprise.
- Avoid pessimism. Pessimism is a denial of your future. What good can come of it?
- Stay open to change and new possibilities. You are a fine piece of art in the making, and the Master Painter is not yet finished with you.

- Throw your hat firmly into the ring of affirmation. Root out negativity: identify it, communicate about it, and deal with it. Avoid negative people; find friends who approach life in a positive, life-affirming way.

## An Affirmative Attitude Says: "Can Do, Will Do"

Though being hopeful about the future is essential to an affirmative attitude, it isn't enough by itself. Hope is only wishful thinking unless we make an effort to bring about what we hope for. This is to say that an affirmative attitude is one that is oriented toward action. When the question is, "Can we find ways to reduce the negative impact of chronic pain on our sex life?" the answer can not just be "I hope so." Instead, make it a resounding "Yes we can. And we will!"

By *action,* I don't mean on-again, off-again efforts that may quickly peter out to nothing. You need concerted efforts that are committed to creating the most fulfilling sexual relationship possible in light of your chronic pain. Yet, it's important to be realistic: dealing effectively with the problem may sometimes be hard work, though that "work" may often turn out to be a lot of fun. And the efforts you put forth prove their value as you and your partner begin experiencing greater sexual fulfillment.

Realize that true affirmation doesn't falter. If you try something and it doesn't work as well as you had hoped, don't give up. Use the feedback that you received to modify your efforts as necessary, or try a new tack. And keep at it. You've probably heard those stories about the water that eventually wears away the rock—just visit the Grand Canyon and you'll see what truly amazing and beautiful things can be done with steady, determined effort. The key to getting to where you want to go is to keep acting, keep moving forward. If one road is blocked, try another. A prime example is communication. A few well-chosen words can make an enormous difference in helping partners relate to one another in positive ways.

## An Affirmative Attitude is Empowering

Embracing an affirmative attitude enables you to approach Cupid's Challenge by *empowering you* to do something about the problem. The fact that empowerment is central to an affirmative attitude is a direct result of its other three main characteristics:

- Instead of ignoring the problem and pretending that everything is rosy, you *realistically* acknowledge the problem.
- Instead of addressing the problem with powerless pessimism, you approach it with constructive *hope.*
- Instead of becoming mired in wishful thinking, you take thoughtful *action.*

By putting these three characteristics together, you empower yourself to start taking steps to deal effectively with the way chronic pain impinges on your sexual happiness. Your goal, of course, is to achieve success and nothing less. By assuming an affirmative attitude—one that is realistic, hopeful, and geared for concerted action—you are making an enormous step toward that achievement.

---

Cupid's Point

Following these guidelines about attitude helps partners to create a safe and relaxed atmosphere for exploration. Can you see how that, in itself, might help to reduce pain levels? (Hint: think of the physiological effects of stress, such as muscle tension and blood pressure.)

Could agreeing on and following such affirming principles also help to create a sexier mood and increase mutual attraction? Is it a way for partners to show respect for each other? And does treating each other with respect tend to enhance closeness inside and outside of the bedroom?

---

## Your Attitude Toward Your Pain

With this basic idea of what an affirmative attitude is, let's turn to the heart of this discussion by explaining four areas where a positive approach is vital in dealing with Cupid's Challenge.

The first area concerns your attitude toward your recurrent pain. A good way to start addressing this aspect is to ask yourself a question: "How do I usually feel about my pain?"

Think about that for a moment. Do you often feel helpless in the grip of chronic pain? When it arrives, do you seem to be at its mercy as it runs roughshod over you? Does it sometimes make you feel totally defeated? If you answer "yes," you are likely permitting your pain to have control over you. You are allowing it, not you, to be your boss.

Strangely enough, some people apparently prefer taking this kind of attitude toward their chronic pain. Perhaps they want to remain in misery because they somehow have sunk into the familiarity of feeling helpless. Or maybe they like the attention they get from their spouse or other family members. But what a sad tradeoff. They concede their life to pain and its attendant limitations just because they are able to complain about it or get to be the center of attention. What they and their enablers don't understand is that they choose their pain if they choose to do nothing about it.

I very much doubt this describes you. Otherwise, you wouldn't be reading this book. The fact that you are is good evidence that you want to take greater control of both your pain and your sex life. It's good evidence that you want to be the one in charge of your pain—not your pain in charge of you.

By embracing such an attitude, you refuse to allow yourself to be defined by your pain. Instead, you adopt an affirmative attitude toward it. At the same time, you step into your proper role as the primary manager of your chronic pain. If you didn't take such a stand, the pain would be unchallenged. But when you do take that stand, the pain meets its match—YOU.

Certainly it's not always easy to embrace such a viewpoint, especially when the pain is acutely present. That's because pain has a tendency, particularly when severe, to make us feel like pawns in its excruciating game. So there may be times when the degree of or the persistence of your pain seriously challenges you for control.

At such times it's wise to have some psychological and behavioral pain management tools handy to help you reduce the intensity of your discomfort or to accept it with more tranquility. By helping you manage your pain, these tools can also assist you in maintaining an affirmative attitude that keeps you moving in the right direction.

Let's briefly examine some non-pharmacological tools that can help you maintain the right mental track as you deal with recurrent pain.

### Self-talk Psychology

What you say to yourself about your pain is a key to helping you develop an affirmative attitude toward managing your pain. Statements that you make out loud or just in your mind such as "I can't stand this," "This pain is horrible," or "I'm never going to get better" promote feelings of helplessness. Consistently replacing such dramatically negative statements with positive ones such as "This pain may be rough, but I can handle it," or "I'm going to get better and better at managing these headaches" can make an immense difference in your attitude.

Using affirmative statements to describe your pain can also lessen the discomfort and intensity of the experience. That's because what you say to yourself about your pain tends to be a kind of self-fulfilling prophecy. Telling yourself it's bad often contributes to making it worse. Telling yourself it's not so bad and that you can handle it though fosters making it easier to handle. It is not that self-talk is a cure-all for pain. Far from it. But it is a potentially powerful tool that you can always have with you in your pain management toolbox.

Cupid's Point

Over several pain incidents, pay attention to what you think and say about the experiences while they're happening and record those statements in a journal as they occur. Afterward, analyze the statements to find out what you are telling yourself about your pain and your ability to cope with it.

If the statements are negative, begin consciously replacing them with more positive, can-do statements when new pain incidents occur. Do these help to make the pain more bearable? Even if not at first, still keep at it. Give the method a chance to work, as it does for so many.

## Biofeedback Therapy

Biofeedback has been found to be useful for alleviating pain caused by a number of conditions, including reflex sympathetic dystrophy (RSD), arthritis, chronic fatigue syndrome, and fibromyalgia, to name a few. This therapy is probably best learned under the guidance of an expert in the method. It involves using an indicator that monitors some changeable bodily state, such as temperature, skin responses, pulse rate, or brain waves. A signal such as a beep is emitted when the state exceeds some desired level. Upon receiving the signal, the user then consciously attempts—for example, by relaxing—to modify the state so that it falls back into the acceptable range.

Biofeedback might more accurately be called *biocontrol,* because that's really what it's all about. You are, via feedback, learning to control certain states of your body, such as brainwaves, that you may not have previously realized you had access to.

Plus, applying biofeedback to control conditions that give rise to pain can make your all-important affirmative attitude even stronger. It does this by showing you can have greater control of your body's states than you may have known, and that you really can learn to manage your pain in significant ways.

### Relaxation Therapy

Stress and pain often go together. For example, many muscle-related conditions and various kinds of headaches are exacerbated by anxiety and stressful experiences. By reducing stress, relaxation strategies can serve as effective tools to help alleviate stress-related pain.

There are many ways to relax, but in dealing with chronic pain it can help if you have a definite set of steps to follow. Progressive muscle relaxation is one option. It begins with finding a comfortable position, usually lying on your back or sitting in an amenable chair. Wait until you are breathing easily and steadily. From that point, professional therapists use different treatment strategies. A common one is to begin by mentally focusing on a specific area of your body for a few breaths as you first tighten your muscles there, then allow them to relax. You may then mentally move to different parts of your body and repeat the same process, spending a little time at each location. This is an especially simple exercise to do. You may even want to take a moment to try it right now.

Progressive muscle relaxation can be seen as a form of biofeedback because it helps you to become more consciously aware of the difference between a tight muscle and a relaxed muscle. This, in turn, helps you to be more aware of when one or more of your muscles are excessively tensed up, and thus be better able to change that state by mentally focusing on relaxing those muscles.

Relaxation therapy can also help keep your attitude working for you. Stress tends to muddy our minds and make our problems seem more difficult. Stress reduction though helps to clear the mental atmosphere so that you can view your situation in a more positive light.

It's important to realize that one main source of the stress that people experience with chronic pain comes from mentally fighting their pain. For instance, mental opposition can express itself physiologically through tensed muscles, which can make the pain even worse. Don't fight against your pain emotionally. Though this may sound contradictory, try to relax with your pain. When it's there, accept the fact that it's there. Mentally relax as best you can. In many cases, this in itself can result in lessening the pain.

## Visualization

Visualization can be used in a couple of different ways as a pain management method. One is to directly visualize the painful part in a way that tends to counteract the pain experience. For example, if the pain in some point of your body feels searingly hot, you could imagine that part as being bathed in cool water. Or if the pain from a headache is associated with some area feeling tight and constricted, you may visualize that area as loosening up and relaxing.

Visualization can also be used as a relaxation tool by helping you get your mind on something other than the pain. A way to do this when pain is present is to assume a comfortable position and then mentally envision a pleasant scenario. This could be imagery of an especially enjoyable experience from your childhood or some delightful place you once visited, perhaps on a holiday. Or it might be some imaginary place or landscape that seems idyllic to you.

Try to fill out the experience or the place you are thinking about in as much detail as possible, bringing all five senses into play. If it's a tropical island scene you're envisioning, then don't forget to see the vivid colors of the birds and smell of the luxuriously fragrant flowers. As you stroll along your imaginary beach, listen to the calming sound of the ocean surf, feel the warm sand beneath your feet, and taste the luscious melon in your hand. This imaginative effort can help counteract the reality of the painfulness.

## Yoga

Yoga is an ancient practice that originated in the Far East thousands of years ago. Today, many find it to be useful for chronic pain management and stress reduction, as well as for increasing body tone and flexibility. There are many forms of yoga, but probably the most useful for the chronic pain survivor are those that focus on combining physical exercises with mental disciplines that conduce to relaxation and serenity.

By emphasizing meditation, calmness, relaxation, and easy breathing, yoga serves as a great antidote to stress and stress-related pain. Though it can be practiced alone, it's probably a good idea to begin your yoga practice with a knowledgeable instructor. The sociability that comes from learning and practicing yoga with others can also strengthen your positive stance toward managing your chronic pain.

Another benefit of yoga is that it can be practiced by individuals at virtually all fitness levels. Though yoga typically includes certain standing, sitting, and lying positions and postures, you do not need to move into any of these that creates considerable discomfort or aggravates your pain. In many cases, the greater flexibility and body tone that arise from yoga practice can also help reduce pain levels. It provides great health benefits too by improving conditioning—and any form of conditioning is better than being sedentary.

Other non-pharmacological methods that you may find useful for managing your pain and increasing your affirmative attitude include:

- Autogenic training—the use of self-hypnosis to create relaxed body states.
- Hypnotherapy—the use of hypnosis to alleviate painful symptoms.
- Massage therapy—massaging the body to relax muscles, increase circulation, and/or balance the body's vital energies.
- Tai Chi—a system of coordinated Chinese exercises.
- Pilates—a system of non-weight-bearing or non-impact exercises to strengthen weaker muscles.
- Acupuncture and acupressure—the use of fine needles, fingers, or blunt instruments at certain points of the body to alleviate pain.

I encourage you to investigate any of these methods that you feel may be of some benefit. However, as always, I strongly suggest you discuss with your physician the advisability, for your particular situation, of any method or regimen that you may be considering before actually engaging in it.

A quick review. Two points became abundantly clear in this section. First, your attitude toward your chronic pain should be an affirmative, empowering one. This is the attitude in which you consistently view yourself not as a victim, but as the active primary manager of your condition and your pain. By assuming a positive view of your ability to manage your chronic pain, you help empower yourself to deal more effectively with it, and thereby with Cupid's Challenge. Here's one way to remember it: Never a victim; always a victor.

Second, there are many non-pharmacological tools out there for you to use as you take on your proper pain management role. Some of these will be more valuable to you than others. But you won't learn which ones work the best for you if you don't investigate them and start putting together your own special chronic pain management toolbox.

## Your Attitude Toward Sex and Your Sexuality

The second area where it's crucial to embrace an affirmative outlook as you confront Cupid's Challenge is in regard to sex and your sexuality. But does this really need to be said? If a couple wants a happier sex life, doesn't it follow that they already have the right attitude toward sex?

Not at all. Partners may desire greater sexual happiness, but at the same time their attitude toward sex or their own sexuality, or possibly both, may be factors preventing them from fulfilling that desire. There are several ways this can happen.

### Two Models of Sexual Activity

First, lovers' attitudes toward sex may differ so greatly that they are not really together when they make love. There is a special danger of this occurring when what the woman wants out of a sexual encounter differs significantly from what the man wants.

Often, a woman's idea of good sex will include a relatively long preliminary period of kissing and caressing that leads eventually to intercourse. Afterwards, some time spent holding, cuddling, and exchanging endearing words may be the ultimate for her. Though this general scenario certainly doesn't describe what all women in our society desire in every sexual encounter, it is the romantic ideal for many women much of the time. It serves to combine romance, seduction, mutual appreciation, intimate physical contact, and a nurturing aspect in the loving tempo of an encounter with several fairly clear-cut stages. Let's call this the *Seduction-Physical Intimacy-Nurturing* (or *SPIN*) model of what a sexual encounter ideally is for many women.

Now, the man's idea of what sex is all about and what he wants out of a sexual encounter may be quite different from his partner's. In particular, men are frequently more goal-oriented in sex than women. And often, the goal is simply to achieve, as quickly as possible, intercourse that leads to ejaculation. Again, there are a lot of men for whom this scenario does not apply well. In particular, there are many men who often, or always, in their feelings and their actions, also relish the SPIN model. However, notoriously, there are many more men for whom the thought of a long, luxurious sexual encounter with their mate is an idea that seldom, if ever, occurs. Furthermore, these days, there is a growing number of women, usually fairly young, whether single or divorced, who seem to emulate men in this respect. These individuals have what we can call the *Goal-Oriented Physical Intimacy* (*GOPI*) model of sexual encounters.

When partners differ in whether they prefer the SPIN or the GOPI type of sexual encounter, a great deal of friction can result. And not the good kind! The woman who thinks in terms of the Seduction-Physical Intimacy-Nurturing model may feel she is being shortchanged by her mate if he acts only according to the Goal-Oriented model. Though she may receive some physical gratification from him and may even achieve orgasm, the all-important romantic and nurturing aspects that she desires go unfulfilled. As this continues over time, she may eventually conclude that her mate neither understands nor appreciates her. She may even start feeling less desire for sex with her partner, which may lead to diminished sexual responsiveness and activity. These changes may also be associated with various negative emotions, such as anger, frustration, anxiety, disappointment, and regret.

---

Cupid's Point

Talk with your partner and decide which of the two models, SPIN or GOPI, each of you tends to prefer—if either. Maybe you will find that there is some third model closer to what one or both of you favor. Or that sometimes you or your partner prefers SPIN and sometimes GOPI.

Discuss what activities you look forward to when thinking about engaging in sex. Be specific. You may learn some important insights about one another. The conversation may also produce considerable heat!

---

For his part, the man in this kind of relationship may feel that his masculinity is being challenged if his partner starts showing him, in one way or another, that he is not satisfying her needs. Instead of reacting in a positive way by trying to learn what those needs are and how he can better fulfill them, he may withdraw to some degree from their sexual relationship. And when they do have sex, he, like his partner, may enjoy it less.

Such fundamental differences about sexual relations are all too common among couples. Now, add chronic pain to the mix and the possibilities for misunderstanding and failing to engage with each other are increased. In fact, because chronic pain brings its own tough challenges to the relationship, its presence is all the more reason for the couple to find a way to get on the same wavelength in their lovemaking.

If divergent attitudes toward what is most pleasurable in sex is something that plagues you and your partner, then a few good doses of something you will learn more about in an upcoming chapter—clear, caring communication—may go a long way toward bringing the two of you closer. Make that communication a priority. Talk with each other in heartfelt language about what you really want out of your sexual relationship. Discuss your differences and what steps you can and will take to draw closer in your mutual approach to your encounters.

As a result of your conversations, you may decide that both of you will try to change your viewpoints somewhat. However, it's likely that the man—at least if he embodies only the goal-oriented model—will need to change more. That's because the Seduction-Physical Intimacy-Nurturing way of relating encompasses much more than the goal-oriented way, and it also is a richer path for joining together sexually.

The upcoming chapters on Touch, Romance, and Innovation focus on helping partners dealing with chronic pain to better relate to one another sexually so they can go far beyond the goal-oriented model. In those chapters you will find plenty of ideas that you and your mate can discuss or try out as you work toward a common attitude concerning your sexual relations. Ideas to help you and your partner to go ahead and take a SPIN!

### Affirm Sex as Worth the Effort

A second way that attitude toward sex and sexuality can hinder a couple in dealing with Cupid's Challenge is by their decision, even if unspoken, that sex just isn't worth the effort. If chronic pain has made sexual relations difficult for the couple in the past, and especially if there are other sexual problems in their relationship, they may conclude that too much effort and energy is required to make things better.

If you ever sometimes wonder whether sex is worth the effort, I hope you'll quickly reassure yourself that the answer is YES. Sex is an extremely important aspect of most of our lives. It is through a couple's sexual encounters that they generally achieve their closest connection and greatest intimacy. If we seldom or never engage in sex with our mate, then a main resource for increasing the depth and satisfaction of our relationship goes largely untapped, and the quality of our lives is lessened. Not to mention that by abstaining from sex with our partner, we miss out on a lot of exquisite pleasure and an excellent tool for combating chronic pain.

In sum, moving toward sexual happiness is almost always worth the effort. And besides, all matters of great value take some energy and discipline to bring about. As you address Cupid's Challenge, cultivate an attitude that sees sexual happiness as a goal well worth striving for. To do otherwise is simply to throw in the towel. And it's way too early for that!

Remember, an affirmative attitude toward improving your sex life is an attitude that is realistic but doesn't get bogged down in those realities. It is also hopeful, forward looking, and action-oriented. I hope that every day you will consciously renew your vision for a more fulfilling sexual relationship. Then focus on how to achieve that vision. And don't forget, any step forward, no matter how small, is an advance.

---

### Cupid's Point

Make a list of all the benefits you do get, used to get, or would get from a satisfying sexual relationship with your partner. What are the physical benefits? The psychological? What are the advantages to your relationship? Are there any spiritual benefits?

Would such a relationship make you better able to manage your chronic pain? How? For even more insights, ask your partner to complete a similar list, then compare notes.

---

Affirm Your Sexuality

A third way your attitude toward sex and sexuality can get in your way is related to the reality that chronic pain is not sexy. In fact, it's about the most unsexy thing around. As a result, those who define themselves by their pain can have a hard time feeling sexy. Remember Karen from an earlier chapter? Her idea of herself as a sexual being was distorted by how she thought a potential partner might view her because she would have to be careful. She couldn't see herself as an attractive, sexy woman if she had to "tiptoe around" in bed. Something like that also seemed to be affecting Ron, the man we met in this chapter. He defined his sexual persona solely on the basis of recent past performances.

But why should Karen or Ron define themselves by their pain, what they have difficulty doing, or past performance? What's to keep Karen from defining herself by her femininity and Ron from defining himself by his masculinity? And what's to keep both of them from defining themselves by what they *can* do?

For most adults, sexual attractiveness has a great deal to do with attitude. I think that the great majority of us would agree that the most attractive members of the opposite sex are usually not the ones with faces or bodies that fit the current cultural norms of "perfection." Rather, sexual attractiveness has more to do with self-confidence, positive interest in the other person, and perhaps a little twinkle in the eye. But if we focus on what we can't do or have difficulty doing in bed, our thoughts will be directed negatively on ourselves instead of positively on the other person. We'll also probably lack that twinkle.

So don't do it. Don't let your pain or disability determine who you feel yourself to be in bed. You are a sexual being, and that's true whether you are afflicted by pain or not. Choose to embrace your sexuality, not the pain.

Likewise, if your partner is living with chronic pain, don't let that define your view of him or her. Behind the pain and whatever disability is causing it, stands the same person you were attracted to years ago. Look past the pain and the behavior associated with it to reveal that person. Your sexy partner is still there, perhaps hiding in the background. Bring him or her out into the forefront again with your loving regard.

## Your Overall Attitude Toward Yourself

The last two sections focused on the importance of affirming yourself in relation to your pain and your sexuality. However, your self-affirmation should not stop there. It will encompass all aspects of your being. In particular, I hope it will include an overall view of yourself as a unique individual with a singular combination of talents and gifts to offer your partner, your family, your friends, and the world.

As the years go by, many of us, whether we have to deal with chronic pain or not, lose sight of how one of a kind we each are. When you were a child, you may have recognized your unique promise. But as you moved through life and confronted various challenges and problems—sometimes successfully and probably sometimes not—your youthful sense of possibility may have diminished.

But those possibilities, whatever they may be in your case, are still very much within you. The first step to beginning to actualize them is to acknowledge that you are still a singular, exceptional creation. And many of the promises that were there when you were younger still remain, waiting to be realized.

What does this have to do with Cupid's Challenge? A lot. By developing a healthy view of yourself as a unique person full of your own special talents and potentialities, you strengthen your inner drive to realize those potentialities. At the same time, you take up a very powerful weapon and don heavy armor for dealing with whatever challenges may arise in your life.

The weapon and the armor are so strong because your healthy sense of self is one of the most powerful forces in nature. When you have a strong sense of who you are, your entire approach to life and its challenges is radically affected.

- You are convinced that you can overcome any problem you face.
- You refuse to admit defeat, even in the most dire circumstances.
- You understand that what happened yesterday doesn't determine what will happen today or tomorrow. For you, the future is always open.
- You realize that the future is determined as much by mental forces, such as attitude, desire, and will, as by physical forces. In fact, you know that in many cases the mental is actually stronger than the physical.

With results like these, no wonder a strong sense of your worth enables you to confront Cupid's Challenge with power!

Is your sense of yourself strong and healthy? Or does it sometimes seem a little anemic? If the latter, a good place to start is spending some quality time figuring out just what your sense of self is at this point in your life. In all likelihood, somewhere inside you is a strong belief in your worth, your unique qualities, and your possibilities even if that view may have been obscured by the toils and challenges of everyday life.

I hope though you will look deep inside and let the truth of who you are reveal itself. You are a special person with your own individual gifts, and you are far stronger than you have probably ever realized. Allow that person who you truly are to bloom in all your beauty and strength. Then let that be the person who confronts Cupid's Challenge.

## Your Attitude Toward Your Partnership

Another area where embracing an affirmative attitude is crucial when confronting Cupid's Challenge involves your view of your partnership. In addressing this issue, it can be useful to start by asking yourself a few simple questions: How do you feel about your partnership? Are you and your partner really together? Or are you walking down separate paths that are diverging more and more?

Those questions are important because, as vital as it is, sex is only one part of your relationship. If other key aspects are not going well, that can create a negative attitude toward the relationship as a whole, which can then make it even more difficult for you to find sexual fulfillment with one another.

Accordingly, as you and your mate confront Cupid's Challenge, also work together to understand and resolve any serious problems other than the chronic pain issues that may be affecting your relationship. In doing so, you can strive to develop a mutually affirmative attitude toward your partnership. As you progress, you will find more avenues to help you and your mate draw closer not only in the bedroom but in other aspects of your lives.

It is important to acknowledge that if partners have been drifting apart for some time, drawing closer can take genuine love for one another, a commitment to making things better, courage, and a lot of communication. Clear, caring communication about issues that may be troubling a relationship, and a belief in the worth of the partnership and of each other, can lead a couple's pathway to start converging again, to start feeling they are walking down the road of life together again.

Everyone loves a story with a happy ending. Make up your mind that you and your partner are going to be the heroes of just such a story. Then keep taking that winning attitude into the bedroom with you as you continue developing your wonderful romantic adventure.

# Chapter Six

# The Arrow of Light

Having to deal with chronic pain can sometimes create a weighty pall in the bedroom. If frustrations mount, the couple may find themselves setting their jaws hard as they attempt to deal with the problem. As a result, the bedroom atmosphere is likely to take on an even more somber cast as the partners grimly forge ahead to achieve sexual happiness.

Hold on just a minute—what was that again? "Grimly forge ahead to achieve sexual happiness." That sounds like an oxymoron—a contradiction in terms!

And of course it is. Couples who find themselves in such a predicament—couples for whom dealing with Cupid's Challenge has become a "very serious issue" in the bedroom—would do well to pause for a moment and contemplate the nature of erotic love. In particular, they should remember that Cupid is a frisky and flirtatious fellow who doesn't flourish well in a gloomy environment. Certainly, chronic pain is a serious issue. But to allow a solemn attitude to invade bedroom activities works against the goal of achieving greater sexual delight. By addressing the problem with such grim determination, the partners unwittingly and ironically create an environment that serves to sabotage, rather than to reinforce their efforts.

The lesson is plain: When addressing Cupid's Challenge, it's crucial for partners to stay not only positive, but also light in their approach. Heaviness versus lightness is a further dimension of attitude, one so important that it deserves its own discussion. Accordingly, in this chapter you will learn how a heavy attitude can arise in the bedroom and why such an approach tends to exacerbate problems. More importantly, you will discover how to cultivate lightness as you confront Cupid's Challenge. In doing so, you will be equipping yourself with yet another of Cupid's superb tools—The Arrow of Light.

## Definitions: Heavy Versus Light

By a *heavy* attitude, I mean one that's characterized by extreme seriousness. When partners display a grave, sober, and humorless approach to Cupid's Challenge, they are assuming a heavy attitude toward the problem. As a result, their approach to sex itself is likely to become inappropriately somber and heavy-minded.

The natural antidote to such extreme seriousness is both powerful and easy to take. It is, simply, to lighten up—to cultivate a light attitude in dealing with Cupid's Challenge. I'm not saying that partners should make light of the challenge itself. Rather, they should be light in the sense of taking a relaxed, accepting, and playful approach to sex.

We can better understand the essence of such a light attitude and how to achieve it by examining more closely how a heavy approach in the bedroom can arise for a couple. As with so many other important issues in life, the better we understand the problem, the more likely we can avoid it.

## Sources of Heaviness

Heaviness in the bedroom can arise in several ways. Three of the most frequent sources are a sense of alienation between partners, a negative attitude, and pressure to perform.

Cupid's Point

What factors other than the ones I mentioned in the text can make for too serious a mood in the bedroom? Do any of the following ever dim the love light for you and your partner?

- Physical or mental tiredness
- Effects of medications
- Worry about non-relationship issues such as finances
- Inability to relax because of pressing obligations

If so, what specific things might you do to deal with the circumstance and create a lighter atmosphere? For example, if medications are making it difficult to lighten up in bed, you could talk to your doctor about taking a pharmaceutical "holiday" or changing your medication. What else?

## Alienation Issues

One common cause of an overly serious approach to sex is some degree of alienation between partners. Unresolved difficulties in a couple's relationship can cast a dark shadow on their efforts to come together in a fulfilling sexual relationship. It's hard to join together in pleasure while feeling separated from one another. Instead of being enjoyable to the partners, sex may feel like a heavy burden to one or both of them.

If this is the source of feelings of heaviness in a couple's bedroom, they are facing a challenge to their relationship that goes beyond chronic pain. And even if the pain issue is satisfactorily resolved, the partners' sex life may remain less than what it once was and what it might again become. Improved communication is a priority for such couples. In particular, they would be wise to form a communication partnership as explained in the next chapter. This can help them address not only how chronic pain is affecting their sex life, but also how other issues are impacting their partnership.

It's also important for them to understand that unresolved relationship difficulties and chronic pain can be interrelated. For example, the stress caused by alienation may intensify and lengthen chronic pain episodes. This is all the more reason why couples who are facing alienation issues should strive to identify their specific problems and work through them. If they are unable to resolve the difficulties on their own, marital counseling may be in order.

## A Negative Attitude

Another main instigator of a too serious approach to sex among partners facing Cupid's Challenge is the absence of faith that their efforts will be successful. If one or both partners approach the problem feeling that they're involved in a hopeless undertaking, then any efforts they make to ameliorate the difficulties may amount to nothing more than going through the motions.

We learned about the importance of maintaining an affirmative attitude in the last chapter. When partners assume such an attitude, they also tend to create a happier, lighter atmosphere in the bedroom. Their belief that they can do something about the way chronic pain affects their sex life helps create a positively uplifting environment— the kind of place where Cupid can breathe easily and show his best stuff. Here again, the critical importance of partners taking an affirmative, empowering approach to whatever problems they may be facing becomes clear.

## Pressure to Perform

A third source of an overly serious approach in the bedroom is a perceived pressure to perform. This widespread cause of a heavy bedroom atmosphere is illustrated clearly by the case of Melissa and Karl, a married couple in their late twenties who faced a major challenge to their sex life when Melissa developed severe arthritis in her hips and knees.

## Melissa and Karl's Story

*To their credit, Melissa and Karl were doing their best to deal with the challenge of chronic pain on their sex life. They discussed the issues openly and made it a point to attempt sex at least once a week as they sought positions and ways of approaching the problem that would get them back on track. So far, however, they had not had much success.*

*It was Saturday night and the couple had made a nine thirty bedroom date to try again. However, both of them had doubts that they would have any more success that night than at other recent times. As the two watched a TV program, Melissa became increasingly apprehensive about their special date. She had taken her medications a little while earlier and so felt little discomfort in her knees and hips. Still, she had no faith that the pain would not flare up once they were in bed.*

*Karl was equally worried. It had been so long since he had pleased Melissa sexually that he wondered whether he would be able to do so that night.*

*At nine o'clock, Melissa went to bathe, and then she retired to the bedroom where she donned a sheer negligee that Karl had bought her for Christmas. She lay down in bed carefully, noting that the discomfort from her movements was minimal.* It had better stay that way, she thought. It had been far too long since she and Karl had had a truly happy sexual encounter. She told herself, we must find a way that night to regain some of the pleasures we used to enjoy. Tonight, the pain just had to stay at bay.

*After his own brief shower, Karl came in and joined his wife.*

*"How are you feeling?" he said, carefully caressing Melissa's left hip over her negligee.*

*"My joints don't feel too bad," Melissa replied. "Maybe this time it will be okay. I really want it to go well."*

*"Me too," said Karl. "We have to find a way to get this right. Our entire sex life is on the line here."*

*"Well, I'm trying the best I can," said Melissa, suddenly tense.*

*"I wasn't saying you aren't. I'm just worried about us."*

*"I'm worried too. But it sounds like you're almost ready to give up."*

*"Why do you say that?" Karl said in a hurt tone. "I'm trying the best I can too."*

*"I know you are, but ..." She tried to see Karl's face in the dim light. As she did so, her hip gave a painful twinge.*

*"No!" she said. "It feels like somebody just stuck a screwdriver into my hip bone."*

*"Don't look at me," Karl said defensively. "Didn't you take your pills?"*

*"Of course I took them." She pushed Karl's hand away and replaced it with her own. As she rubbed her hip, she continued, "It's the same every time. On the nights when we try, we start arguing as soon as we get into bed. Half the time we don't even get started."*

*"I know," Karl said. "It spoils the mood immediately." After a moment he continued, "You're obviously not ready for anything. Nor am I. Let's just go to sleep."*

*Melissa agreed, though with the uncomfortable realization that this time they had given up more quickly than ever before.*

Can you feel it? The heavy atmosphere in Melissa and Karl's bedroom is almost palpable. It began with their excessive anxiety about how the evening would turn out as they let past defeats spread a drab mood over present attempts. In doing so, they neglected to follow a principle that we learned in the last chapter—Don't Get Bogged Down in the Past. Don't let your self-image or your present efforts be defined by past difficulties or negative experiences just as Melissa and Karl fell prey to the mistake of letting their past sabotage their present.

One root cause of the heavy mood surrounding Karl and Melissa was that they brought to bed an attitude of "Do or Die"—the idea that they *had* to get it right this time. This extreme self-applied pressure added to their self-doubts and created a tension that got their communication off on the wrong track almost immediately. Then, when Melissa felt a twinge of pain, it took only a moment before they decided to call it quits for the night.

Karl and Melissa's case clearly illustrates the very negative effects that can result when one or both partners feel great pressure as they address Cupid's Challenge. The pressure they feel is to perform, to get it right, to make it happen. It's the pressure to "enjoy sex, dammit!" And in this characterization we can see how absurd it is.

When we feel pressure to perform, it may or may not come partly from our mate. But in every case, it largely, if not entirely arises from ourself. That's because no matter what our partner says or doesn't say, we have to buy in to the idea that we must perform. In the final analysis, it's the individual alone who puts demands on him or herself.

Unfortunately, when we do put pressure on ourselves, we sometimes end up mistakenly accusing the other person of pressuring us. This is what happened in Karl and Melissa's case. When we look at their thoughts, it becomes clear that the heaviness each partner felt was being self-applied. But then each of them became so sensitive to the other's words that they accused one another of putting pressure on them. And when that started happening, their date quickly fell apart.

The heavy demands that we put on ourselves typically come from our desire to live up to some idea of what we must be able to do if we are to "perform" well. Examples of such requirements are to:

- Get through the night without pain.
- Achieve an orgasm.
- Please my partner.
- Do what I once was able to do.
- Make everything right tonight!

The pressure typically takes the form of mental statements that we are often barely conscious of; statements such as:

- If I don't get this right, she (or he) won't love (or respect or appreciate) me any more.
- My pain just can't flare up again tonight. If it does, that would be terrible!

- My masculinity (or femininity) is on the line. If I'm not able to do this, I'm not a real man (or woman).
- She thinks I don't find her sexy any longer because of her pain. I have to prove to her that's not true.
- He probably doesn't find me sexually desirable because of my pain. I have to prove to him that I am.

All of these statements take the form of self-ultimatums. They all use negative words such as "won't" or "can't" or phrases indicating that the individual *has* to do something to show that he or she is a "real" man or woman, or to "prove" something else. For some people, some of the time, strong self-ultimatums may prove motivationally useful. However, for most of us, most of the time—and especially when sexual fulfillment is the matter at hand—applying such strong self-pressure tends to backfire, as it did with Karl and Melissa.

Presenting strong ultimatums to ourselves about our sexual performance can be counterproductive for any of several reasons. First, if we doubt that we can fulfill whatever the ultimatum requires, we will likely become anxious. The anxiety arises because we are telling ourselves two things—that we have to succeed, and that we will probably fail. This is not a message destined to increase our libido!

Second, we may project the source of the ultimatum onto our partner. We start thinking that it's the other person who is making the demand on us, when it's actually only ourselves. That's what happened to Karl and Melissa when they started viewing each other as the source of a demand that they were each applying only to themselves.

Third, putting severe pressure on ourselves creates a kind of heaviness of mind, emotions, and spirit that is diametrically opposed to sexual enjoyment. The happiest, most fulfilling sex is not heavy at all. It's more like an exciting, enjoyable game.

However, if we lose sight of the true nature of erotic love, it may help if we travel back to our early adulthood and recall what sex was like when it was brand new. So let's do just that. By taking a moment to remember what erotic love was like when we first came of age, we may get a clearer idea of what we to seek out as we deal with Cupid's Challenge.

## Sex as Play

Back then, sex was a wonderful, mysterious, romantic new aspect of our life. Learning about our sensuality and sexuality was an exciting process of discovery that we ideally played with one special partner who was also discovering the secrets of sex.

For many or most of us, our excitement continued through at least the early parts of our marriages. Do you remember what it was like early in your relationship, when all through the day you anticipated being with your partner that evening? Do you recall the times when you spent the day looking forward, not only to a dinner or movie date, but also to arriving back home? Can you still feel the excitement of getting dressed up for that special night out, of making sure your hair was perfectly arranged, or for you guys ensuring that you were cleanly shaven? Do you remember the questions you used to ask yourself— Will he like my lipstick? What kind of flowers should I bring home to her? Is my breath fresh?

What a delicious game it was we played back in those days! And if we played it well, there was not a hint of heaviness to it. It was light, erotic, sensual, and profoundly joyful.

Perhaps you and your partner can never re-experience the precise newness and mystery that sex presented to the two of you in the very beginning. But that doesn't mean you can't recapture, and who knows, maybe even outdo the sense of playfulness and excitement that marked your early sexual experiences! At the very least, you can set before yourselves the ideal of light-hearted and erotically charged sexual experiences as a goal to aim for as you address Cupid's Challenge. To do so requires remaining light in your mind and your approach. And cultivating lightness, in turn, requires a commitment to taking the pressure off yourselves and each other.

---

Cupid's Point

To help refresh your sexual feelings for your partner and renew the excitement that you felt when you first got together, take some time to reflect on what first attracted you to him (or her). What were the attributes that "turned you on" when you were first together— their face, smile, look, smell, voice, eyes, shyness, boldness, ideas, ambition, loyalty?

Make a list of those positive qualities. If you think hard, you may find it to be a rather long one. Which of those same characteristics can you still see in your partner? Are there any that you are now aware of that you didn't see back then?

---

## How to Keep It Light

Fortunately, there are many specific things that you and your partner can do and say to prevent a heavy atmosphere from descending on your bedroom. To gather some ideas, let's revisit Karl and Melissa again.

The couple's evening didn't have to end so precipitously and on such a defeatist note. There were numerous things they could have said to each other to dispel the heaviness that eventually engulfed them. For example, in responding to Melissa's statement "I really want it to go well," Karl could have made a comment expressly meant to defuse the tension, such as:

- "I do too, but let's just take it easy tonight and have fun," or
- "I know we'll get it right eventually. Let's relax and see what happens."

Or he could have made an erotic or appreciative comment, such as:

- "After one look at you in that negligee, my body's telling me it will go very well."
- "Touching you like this is already making me hot."
- "You look great tonight."

Any such statement by Karl invoking a relaxed and accepting attitude would have helped reduce the tension the couple felt from their self-ultimatums to perform. And it certainly would have been preferable to his actual reply, which included the apocalyptic "Our entire sex life is on the line here."

Talk about putting the pressure on! It's no wonder that Cupid would have trouble shooting his arrows straight, given that heavy weight.

Melissa, too, could have made any number of comments to help lighten the "Oh So Serious" mood that stalled their date. It's not that either partner needed to say something wonderfully wise, romantic, or witty to put things into proper perspective. Just a simple "Don't worry, we'll be fine," "You smell good," or "That feels nice," could have immediately helped to calm nerves and change a serious mood to a sexy, hopeful one. Instead of quitting at the first sign of trouble, the lovers would have then been more likely to explore ways to get around Melissa's hip pain.

The main point here is just this: What you and your partner say in bed and how you say it are extremely important. If your words express only disguised or explicit demands on yourself or your partner, or if they express doubts or worries, then don't be surprised if the light, erotic, playful atmosphere that you seek remains elusive. But if your words are accepting, hopeful, appreciative, and relaxed, they will help create the kind of environment in which Cupid thrives.

This can be difficult to remember at the moment when you are being confronted with pain or while the chatter of your mind is getting in your way. That's why it's important for you and your partner to discuss beforehand the importance of taking a light approach in the bedroom. Those talks can help you to do two things: identify and defuse self-ultimatums, and make a firm choice to cultivate a light, relaxed, and playful atmosphere in your sex life.

## Identify and Defuse Self-ultimatums

The first step in dealing with self-ultimatums is for you and your mate to become aware of whether either of you is feeling excessive pressure to perform. In your own case, this will be reflected in your mood and in what you say to yourself, especially in demands that you set for yourself. If your partner is also feeling pressure, he (or she) may not be consciously aware of doing this. Even so, the pressure will probably be reflected in his statements or manner.

If you find that you are feeling the weight of self-ultimatums, then look inside to try to understand what they are. In the next chapter, we will talk about communicating with yourself to find out what you truly feel. That's what you need to do here—articulate clearly to yourself what specific demands you are placing on yourself. If it's your partner who is laboring under self-ultimatums, identify them and get them into words using the principles of communication described in the next chapter to help create a safe place for expression.

In addition, ask yourselves whether either of you feels that the other is expecting too much. Does either partner feel that what is done or not done in bed "proves" something about manhood or womanhood or the attractiveness of either partner?

---

Cupid's Point

To help defuse a self-ultimatum, ask yourself pointed questions about it and pay attention to how difficult it is to provide reasonable answers:

- Why do we have to solve all of our problems tonight? Who decided that schedule?
- Why does my having an orgasm "prove" that I am a "real" man (or woman)? Is this some sort of scientific fact?
- Who says that being subject to chronic pain makes me unsexy? If I say it about myself, what is my basis?

Does it make any sense to put pressure on yourself if doing so gets in the way of enjoying sex? After all, what is your true objective? Is it to prove something about yourself? Or is it to have enjoyable sex with your partner?

---

Once you both understand how ultimatums and judgments may be playing a role in your thoughts and feelings, talk about how to defuse them. Affirm to each other that you are not there to invalidate anything about yourself or the other person. Instead, commit yourselves to the idea that dealing effectively with Cupid's Challenge is about self-acceptance and not about proving anything. It's not a competition, a test, a race, or an exam. It's a matter of the two of you discovering, in your own good time, ways to improve your sexual relationship while also managing chronic pain. Your goal can be to design a less demanding atmosphere where the two of you can relax in the certainty that you are only there to enjoy each other's company.

### Choose to Create a Light, Relaxed Atmosphere

You and your partner will best be able to achieve the kind of light, relaxed atmosphere that is amenable to sexual happiness if you make a clear, conscious commitment to creating that space. Like so many other aspects of facing Cupid's Challenge effectively, this is a matter of choice. Don't expect different results from the same old approach and behavior. Instead of letting your random thoughts and moods dictate your encounter—which is what happened with Karl and Melissa—take the time to consciously create the scenario you prefer. Choose to work with your lover to determine the environment you want to cultivate. Then commit yourselves to creating that environment.

The choice that you make is between the heavy and the light. Do you take a ponderous, heavy-handed approach that is marked by pressure, performance anxieties, and spoken or unspoken ultimatums? Or do you opt for the light, playful, erotic approach that is Cupid's natural way?

Realize that a further important benefit of choosing the light approach is that mental relaxation tends to foster physical relaxation. That, in turn, can often help reduce pain by reducing stress, which is another big plus.

## Understand What Play Is All About

As you and your partner talk about the atmosphere you want to create in your bedroom, it may be helpful to focus more on the concept of play. That's because play has three characteristics that can enhance your lovemaking as you deal with Cupid's Challenge: it's open, explorative, and spontaneous.

As for play being open, think of recreational activities. In those, rules tend to be relatively nonrigid. The participants often make up rules as they go, or change the rules to meet the needs of the occasion. And if someone enters a game insisting on lots of strict, by the book structure, the game tends to become more stultifying and less pleasurable. Of course, a few rules are usually needed. But there shouldn't be too many. It's more fun when someone just draws a line with a foot in the dirt and says, "Here are the boundaries. No double dribble or hard fouling. Now let's play!"

Much the same goes for sex. There need to be a few basics to abide by. Rules that everyone understands. For example, seek your partner's pleasure, let him or her know what feels good, and be loving. Okay, now it's time to play!

Play is also, by its nature, explorative. The importance of exploring your sensuality and sexuality as you address Cupid's Challenge is something you will find highlighted many times in this book; for instance with the *ICE* method in which the third stage is *Explore*. That emphasis on exploration fits right into the idea of sex as playful and light. As you and your lover seek effective ways to improve your sex life despite chronic pain, don't forget the value of exploring your sexuality. Remember that satisfying sexual encounters need not always make intercourse or orgasm as their goal. In your explorations, don't be surprised if you discover some new sexual pleasures—new moves to make in the exciting and rewarding game of sexual discovery.

Finally, play tends to be spontaneous. A little spontaneity can go a long way by making the game of sex doubly delicious—like a refreshing treat when we least expect it.

One way to cultivate spontaneity is for partners to invite each other into sensual get-togethers at appropriate but unaccustomed places or times. This can be an excellent way to refresh sexual taste buds and help restore some excitement. Understand that spontaneity doesn't always have to be totally spontaneous. In the section The Arrow of Romance, we will learn more about planned spontaneity and how it can heighten the intensity of your sexual encounters.

### Don't Make Lightness Heavy

Be careful not to make the idea of being light into an overly serious goal for you and your partner. Lightness should remain light. To help keep it so, remember that what's important as you address Cupid's Challenge is simply that you two are together and that your main objective is just to enjoy each other's company as you move, in a relaxed, nondemanding way toward even greater enjoyment. Partners can help one another to relax by assuring each other of this during their encounters

## Using Humor to Keep It Light

It's the same for sex as for many other aspects of life—the appropriate use of humor can help keep a mood from becoming overly serious and can restore lightness. Make sure that the humor is appropriate, though. In the context of sexual relations, where we tend to be very vulnerable, a backhanded joke can be like a bucket of water thrown on a campfire. Even a small "witticism" at the expense of your lover—regardless if the intention is harmless—can cause a heavy mood to descend very quickly.

After being together for a while, partners usually come to understand what kinds of humor each other responds to positively. Couples often develop a store of private jokes and mutual ways of looking at the world as a funny place that help them bond and create camaraderie. That's the kind of humor that can help you and your lover keep it light in bed.

Humor that shines a funny light on their situation can help partners get through some rough spots too. The right kind of laughter at the right time gives an encounter room to breathe by defusing the power of self-ultimatums and thereby releasing pressure. But remember, it isn't funny unless it's funny for both. And it isn't funny for both unless it makes you both feel lighter inside.

Whatever specific tools you use—humor, loving discussions, appreciative words, gentle touches—lightness should always be one of your main goals as you seek a happier sex life. Think of The Arrow of Light as doing double duty. It helps keep your encounters playful, erotic, and light, while at the same time it helps you and your partner open up any concerns hiding in the shadows that sometimes accompany chronic pain.

The Arrow of Light, being so tied to the essence of erotic love, is one of Cupid's favorites. Be sure to give it a prominent place in your quiver.

# Chapter Seven

# The Arrow of Communication

The importance of good communication in confronting Cupid's Challenge becomes obvious when we list some of the crucial ways it enables couples to:

- Understand how pain is affecting their sex life.
- Understand each other's specific sexual desires.
- Express and release their frustrations.
- Identify specific ways to address Cupid's Challenge.
- Explore their sensuality together.
- Achieve greater intimacy.

However, understanding communication's value is only the first step in making relating well work for you and your partner. To move forward, it's crucial to understand how to communicate effectively. That can be especially difficult with the taboos and embarrassment that often accompany issues surrounding Cupid's Challenge. The kinds of questions my patients ask me sometimes reflect this difficulty:

- Why is it so hard for my spouse and I to discuss problems concerning chronic pain and sex?
- How can we improve our communication about these matters?
- What particular strategies or techniques might make our discussions more productive?

Our goal in this chapter is to get some useful answers to those pressing questions. In particular, we will focus on ideas, principles, and strategies that can help you make The Arrow of Communication one of your most powerful tools as you face the challenge that chronic pain presents to your love life.

A good place to begin is with the question of who it is advisable to communicate with about Cupid's Challenge—because it's not just your partner.

## Communicating with Yourself

When your objective is to effectively communicate with someone else, often the best place to start is to have a good talk with yourself. That's especially true for individuals who may be somewhat out of touch with their deepest feelings. Consider Mary, a woman in her mid-forties who had suffered from stress headaches for years though recently the headaches had begun affecting her sex life with her husband, Charles. But the link between Mary's headaches and the couple's sexual problems didn't become clear until she learned a few things about herself.

### Mary and Charles' Story

*Mary's headaches had typically occurred in the late afternoon or early evening after a long day at work. Usually, they would be gone after a few hours and seldom had any impact on her sexual relations with her husband, Charles. But for the last few months, her headaches had frequently erupted just before bedtime. Though she took a painkiller immediately, it was usually half an hour or more before she felt comfortable. During that period, if Charles made any advances, she gently refused him. And by the time the pain was gone he would be asleep.*

*Mary didn't know why this change had occurred, but she did know that it was playing havoc with her and Charles' love life to the point that her husband was starting to complain. So at her next appointment with her physician, she hesitantly brought up the problem.*

*"Were there any sexual problems before this development?"* Mary's doctor asked.

*"No."*

*"Do you normally enjoy sexual relations with your husband?"*

*"I guess so,"* Mary replied. *"Why do you ask?"*

*"I was exploring the possibility that your headaches might be serving as a way to avoid sex."*

*"What a thing to suggest! You think I'm pretending to have the headaches?"*

*"Not at all,"* her doctor replied. *"I'm sure they are very real, and probably the result of stress. But I was wondering if the stress might be caused by the idea of having sex—whether it might be your body's way of helping you to avoid intimacy."*

*"Well, that's certainly not the problem in my case,"* she answered indignantly.

*Later, at home, Mary kept thinking about what her doctor had suggested. Surely there couldn't be anything to it. But slowly she started realizing that actually most of the time she didn't really enjoy sex any longer. Somehow, without her really being consciously aware of it, sex had evolved into a duty thing, a duty that she no longer wanted to perform.*

*This was a revelation to Mary. How could she have felt this way for so long and not have realized it? The truth had been there, hidden beneath the surface, but it had not been communicated to her conscious mind. Only her doctor's questioning and her subsequent questioning of herself had brought Mary to realize an important insight.*

*This realization didn't solve Mary and Charles' problem, but it was a necessary first step to a solution. It set Mary looking for the reasons for her change in feelings, which fostered even more effective self-communication. Once those reasons were identified—which revolved around Mary's growing belief that Charles didn't appreciate her—she and her husband were able to talk honestly about their feelings. The result of several difficult but rewarding discussions between the two was a better understanding of each other and a commitment to work on renewing their sexual bond.*

Mary's case illustrates a kind of situation that is quite common—a place in life where we are out of touch with our true emotions or beliefs. Something deep inside is not being clearly communicated to our conscious mind. And because the truth is not represented clearly in our consciousness, it can't be clearly articulated in our thoughts or in our words when we talk to others—particularly those we are intimate with.

This kind of disconnection between our feelings and our understanding of them might occur for any number of reasons. What we truly feel may seem to contradict our self-image. Or there may be a sense of guilt associated with our deep emotions. Or it may simply be difficult for us to know what we feel because we haven't taken the time to try to understand what that is.

Whatever the reason, the truth can sometimes be hidden for a long time. Mary had failed for several months to recognize how her feelings about having sex with her husband had changed. During that time, her headaches, brought on by the stress of facing something she had come to dread, had helped keep her from having to engage sexually. Once she understood those feelings, she was able to communicate them to her husband. Without that first key step, she and Charles would have been unable to understand and effectively address the real problem.

As you and your partner face Cupid's Challenge, keep Mary's case in mind. None of us can articulate our own feelings perfectly, and becoming fully conscious of those feelings can be hard work. But it's important for you both to understand as well as possible how each of you truly feels about the way chronic pain is affecting your sex life.

Here are some questions to ask as you probe your feelings:

- How do I feel about my current sexual relations with my partner? Do I enjoy them? Are there certain aspects of those relations that I like and others that I don't like as much, or that I definitely dislike?

- How do I feel about my partner? Do I think that he or she approaches me with enough affection, respect, consideration, and desire? During sex, does he or she behave in some ways that particularly please me? Or displease me?

- What, if anything, would I like to change about our sex life? Would I like to alter some aspects of what we actually engage in? Or the frequency or duration of our encounters? Do I experience enough emotional closeness with my partner during sex?

- How do I feel about my (or my partner's) chronic pain or disability in relation to our sex life? Do I attempt to cover over the pain or disability? Or try to ignore it? What specific problems does it cause? Are these just physical problems, or are they also emotional or psychological problems? Do I feel that we are dealing effectively with those issues?

Addressing these questions can be a valuable exercise by way of examining your deep thoughts and emotions and allowing them to rise to your conscious mind where you will be better able to clearly articulate yourself. Ideally, your partner will also try to understand his or her feelings about your sexual relations and how chronic pain affects your intimacy.

There are several methods that can help you clarify your true feelings. One is to try to capture them on paper, for instance in a journal. The inner truth gets transformed into physical marks on a sheet of paper that you can see right in front of your eyes. As you then read and think about the words you have written, ask yourself whether they adequately represent what you feel. If not, probe deeper and revise your writings until they express your thoughts and emotions accurately.

An even simpler way of trying to understand your feelings is to relax in a comfortable chair or on your bed while you ask yourself specific questions such as those listed above. Ask yourself what you genuinely think about a particular issue. Take your time and let your feelings speak for themselves. Articulate, aloud or silently, your answer to each question. Then ask yourself, "Is there more I need to understand here?" If so, search more deeply.

Both of these methods are simple to perform. Yet amazingly, countless important dialogues transpire each day in which the participants enter into the conversation without spending even a few minutes beforehand trying to clarify what they really think and feel about the issues to be discussed.

Don't let that happen to you and your partner. Listen to and try to understand the truth inside you. Whatever means you use, strive to create a clear conduit that will allow your deepest thoughts and emotions to be clearly communicated.

## Communicating with Your Physician

Many couples whose sex lives are troubled by chronic pain neglect to make full use of one of their most obvious and useful allies—their physician. They may look to their doctor to help them manage their pain, yet never consider the possibility that he or she might also be able to assist them in dealing with the more specific problem of how that pain affects their sex life.

One reason partners do this is out of embarrassment: they feel awkward bringing the subject up with their doctor. Also, they may not realize that their physician is knowledgeable about how chronic pain can affect all kinds of life functions, including sex. They don't understand what an exceedingly valuable resource their doctor can be as they face Cupid's Challenge.

To make the best use of that resource, clear communication is the key. And that begins with you. Your doctor can't know what problems you are having in the bedroom unless you disclose those problems, so make sure to bring them up at your appointment.

---

**Cupid's Point**

If Cupid's Challenge is affecting your relationship, have you discussed the problem with your physician? If not, take a few minutes to record on paper the specific points you might discuss with your doctor.

Be sure to include all relevant facts about the pain, its effect on your sexual relations, and any role that medications may be playing. Then write down several specific questions that you would like to ask your doctor.

All that's left now is to take your questions to your physician. Don't be shy. Answering your questions is one of the things your doctor is there for.

---

Here are some ideas to help you make the most of your time as you discuss these important issues with your doctor:

Know what you want to say. Appointment times tend to be short these days, so it's important that you go to your meeting with a clearly formulated idea of just what you want to say. That means you should set aside adequate time beforehand to communicate with yourself about what you want to talk to your doctor about. Write it down. Memorize it. Be prepared to tell your doctor briefly and accurately just how chronic pain is affecting your sexual relations—what hurts, how much it hurts, and how, specifically, the pain limits you and your partner. No need to be embarrassed. Your doctor is a professional who is interested only in understanding the medical issues and in providing advice, and/or treatment that may help alleviate difficulties.

Take notes. It's a good idea to bring along a notebook and a pen to your appointment so you can take notes. A tape recorder may be convenient, but be sure to inform your physician before starting. In any event, don't depend on your memory of what your doctor says—record it in some way. This will give you an accurate record to help you relay to your partner any important information you gain from your physician.

Discuss any changes you are considering. Make sure you bring up anything new such as new positions, activities, frequencies, or therapies that you and your lover have been considering to help you deal with Cupid's Challenge. Share these with your doctor and solicit his or her comments. As a rule, always seek your health professional's advice before making any changes that could potentially have harmful health effects.

As a doctor, I can tell you that it is a genuine pleasure for me when a patient comes to my office with a clearly articulated set of questions related to his or her health and wellness. That tells me the patient is taking an active role in managing his or her health. I think the great majority of doctors feel the same way. They appreciate an active, informed patient who communicates.

## Communicating with Your Partner—What Makes it So Hard?

So far, we've discussed communicating with yourself and with your physician about how chronic pain is affecting your sex life. Now we come to the critical subject of communicating effectively with your partner. For many couples that's one of the most troublesome aspects of dealing effectively with Cupid's Challenge.

The first thing we need to understand is why it's often difficult for couples to communicate about issues surrounding chronic pain and sexuality. There can be many reasons, but a few stand out.

Difficulties in discussing sex. You might think that talking about sex would be easy for most anyone these days when sex seems to be a chief commodity sold over our televisions and in many magazines. But for millions, sex remains an embarrassing topic to broach, even with their partner. And it can be especially embarrassing if it involves sexual dysfunction. Our sense of who we are is partly defined by who we feel we are sexually, and to admit that our sex life is not functioning well may feel uncomfortable and threatening.

Difficulties in discussing chronic pain. It can also be difficult for one or both partners to bring up the subject of pain or disability. For instance, the one who bears the pain may feel guilt or embarrassment. He or she may view their chronic pain as creating a burden for the partnership. A problem for the other person may be fear that bringing up the topic will be seen as complaining about, rather than supporting, the partner. If both members of the couple feel hesitant about addressing the topic of chronic pain, the result may be a wall of silence.

The attrition of time. It may be difficult for a couple to discuss their issues surrounding Cupid's Challenge simply because their ability to communicate effectively with one another has eroded over time. This is a problem that affects millions of couples. More specifically, the idea of sitting down and working through a problem affecting their sex life may strike many couples as virtually impossible. Or at least, after years of lackluster communication they may be laced with anger and resentment, and they don't really know where to start.

Different communication styles. Varying communication styles can quickly lead a dialogue astray as well. For example, one partner may be interested only in the cognitive aspects of a problem, wanting to get right down to identifying and talking about the specific elements of the issue. Yet, the other partner may consider the creation of an emotionally warm atmosphere to be a necessary precursor to effective communication. Partners may also differ in other ways that are relevant to their communication such as how much patience they bring to a dialogue, or how aware they are about their own feelings.

Try to become attuned to whatever may hinder your clear communication about Cupid's Challenge. Is it hard for one or both of you to talk about your sex life? Or about the chronic pain that is affecting it? Do you find it difficult to discuss problems without getting impatient or angry with each other? Do your communication styles differ significantly?

If your answer is yes to any of these questions, take heart. There are practical steps that you and your partner can take to reduce or eliminate communication obstacles. These steps start with committing yourselves to clear, caring communication.

## Communication Partnerships

Whatever the issue is being discussed, communication between partners must be a joint project to have a good chance for success. But as we've just seen, many couples dealing with Cupid's Challenge find themselves far apart in their efforts to communicate. Like inhabitants of separate mountain peaks, they call to each other across a gulf so wide that there is little authentic contact. Or worse, they remain silent.

Being together as you communicate doesn't require you and your partner agree on every issue. But the more united you are in your determination to talk things through, the more likely you will be able to formulate effective strategies for improving your sex life.

An excellent way to draw closer together in your communication is to consciously enter into a *communication partnership*. Such a partnership begins with a mutual decision to work together in making your communications as fruitful as possible. You make that decision because you understand that communication is at the foundation of any successful relationship; but you have to work at it. Ideally, your communication partnership will extend to all serious issues that affect your relationship, though it is definitely advisable to enter into such an agreement in regards to Cupid's Challenge.

### Communicating about Communication

Once you decide to enter into a communication partnership, your next natural step is to determine how to make that decision a reality. And that, in turn, requires spending some quality time communicating about the communication process itself. Such a dialogue typically includes two main parts.

The first is to jointly identify and discuss any potential roadblocks that could hinder your efforts to communicate. Here, you may find it helpful to refer back to our discussion earlier in this chapter about what makes it difficult to discuss Cupid's Challenge. Is it a problem for either partner to talk to the other about your sex life or about the chronic pain or disability impinging on it? Has overall communication between the two of you fallen on hard times lately? Do you have different conversational styles that result in your talking at cross-purposes? Addressing these questions can help you identify problems that make it difficult to articulate and discuss the issues effectively so that you can then seek solutions.

Even when a couple is only trying to identify problems that may hinder their talks, they may find themselves butting heads. Which brings us to the second main part of communicating about communication—understand and commit yourselves to sound conversational principles. The better you and your partner grasp the maxims of good communication, the stronger your communication partnership will become. To that end, let's focus on some key principles that help lay the groundwork for great dialogues.

### Five Principles of Good Communication
Talk truthfully. As obvious as this rule may seem, it's violated innumerable times in countless conversations between partners. And I'm not referring here to dialogues in which one person is trying to deceive another. I mean conversations in which both members of the couple want to be truthful but fail to do so for one reason or another. This may be because they are afraid of hurting the other person's feelings, or are embarrassed to speak the truth, or don't understand their own feelings well enough to articulate them. So it is important to understand your true feelings before entering into a dialogue. And don't let a little embarrassment deflect you from saying what you believe to be true.

But what if speaking the truth might hurt your partner's feelings? You can minimize that possibility by the way you express yourself. Realize that honest and brutally honest are two different things. When discussing what are potentially difficult emotional issues, it's important to use gentle, judicious words. At the same time, it's crucial to speak the truth. If the two of you are not prepared to do that, then how can you expect to make any progress in dealing with whatever realities you are facing?

Talk clearly and to the point. It's often easy to get sidetracked when a conversation relates to highly emotional matters, which dialogues concerning Cupid's Challenge often do. So stay calm and don't let your emotions sabotage your communications. Tools for achieving this include trying to be sensitive to whether you are getting off track and reminding each other of what you are trying to accomplish.

As for talking clearly, realize that it can be difficult, both for you and your partner, to articulate your feelings. By getting as clear as possible beforehand about what you think and feel you can express yourself more lucidly. If you don't think your partner is making his or her feelings clear, then ask for clarifications, expansions, and illustrations. But do so gently, gently.

Listen attentively. Attentive listening is one of your most crucial communication skills. Good communication between two people is not unidirectional. It's not one person talking down to, or at, the other. Rather, it's about partners working together to understand each other. That means each person has to be able to have his or her say. You may feel that what you want to communicate to your partner is very important. And it may well be. But don't forget that your partner also has important feelings to communicate. So each should create the space that will allow the other to say what is in their heart.

Being an attentive listener requires learning how to calm the chatter of your mind and focus on your partner's words and their meaning. If, while your partner is trying to express his or her thoughts, you are busy formulating your next comment or wondering whether so-and-so is going to call, then your mate might as well be talking to the walls. And that's not what either of you wants. For the dialogue to go forward, each of you needs to understand what the other has to say. And that only comes through careful, attentive listening.

Keep an open mind. Nothing dampens communication faster than a closed mind. Maintaining an open mind means being willing to listen to what your mate says without ridicule or any other form of emotional negativity. This doesn't mean that you have to agree with what your partner is saying. But if you disagree, make it a cognitive disagreement as much as possible, and keep your emotions at bay. It's okay to say, "I don't see it that way" or "I don't think I would like engaging in that kind of sexual activity" if that's the way you feel. But refrain from "You're wrong!" or "Where did you get such a weird idea?" And even if you don't see it the other person's way at first, keep an open mind. Both participants must believe that the conversation is a safe place to verbalize their ideas and desires.

Support each other in the communication process. Listening attentively and keeping an open mind help you support each other as you communicate. Likewise, talking truthfully and to the point are ways of showing respect for, and in that way supporting, one another.

The support rule makes especially good sense when your dialogue is about Cupid's Challenge. After all, what you and your partner are aiming for is a more fulfilling sexual relationship in the face of chronic pain. And such a relationship is ideally one in which you strongly support each other in your mutual sexual activities. It only makes sense to start moving toward that more intimate and rewarding relationship by supporting each other in your conversations.

Communication support comes in two forms: emotional and cognitive. Emotional support is important because it's easy for partners to feel emotionally vulnerable when the conversation is about how chronic pain affects their sex life. You or your partner may feel somewhat awkward or embarrassed in talking about such issues, or you may fear criticism if you say what you really think. To help short circuit such anxieties, use caring words to make clear to one another that there is nothing to fear in talking openly. This can go a long way toward creating an emotional atmosphere that will allow the two of you to discuss issues honestly.

One of the best ways for you and your partner to emotionally support one another as you discuss Cupid's Challenge is to show your affection and concern for each other. Your conversations are excellent opportunities to express your mutual regard. Assure one another of your love, that *you are in this together,* and that you are there to support each other. By doing so, you help empower your dialogues for maximum success.

Cognitive support is also important. Partners can cognitively support each other in several ways:

- Urge your partner to speak honestly and openly.
- Help your mate to communicate what he or she wants to say by asking for clarifications and examples if there is something you don't understand.
- Don't put words in the other person's mouth and don't jump to conclusions. Listen carefully. Provide the space and time for your partner to say what he or she needs to say.
- To help avoid miscommunication, it's often useful to give feedback on what you believe the other person is saying. You might say, for example, "What I hear you telling me, Dear, is that…" (here you paraphrase your partner's words).
- Be aware of whether your mate seems to understand what you are trying to say. If you think you are not being understood well, try to explain your points or ideas more clearly.

It's good to remember that supporting each other emotionally and cognitively is a way of holding each other closer. That's often a great aphrodisiac in itself and may be a prelude to scintillating sex!

---

**Cupid's Point**

Think about the last few times you and your partner sat down together to discuss some concern. Did you both adhere to all of the principles of good communication mentioned in this chapter? If not, which principles were violated? In what way? Which ones were followed most closely? Least closely?

Would your conversations have been more productive if you had agreed on some communication ground rules beforehand?

---

In sum, you and your lover can give substance to your communication partnership by committing yourselves to Five Principles of Good Communication:

- Talk truthfully.
- Talk clearly and to the point.
- Listen attentively.
- Keep an open mind.
- Support each other as you communicate.

Don't take any of these for granted. Don't assume that you understand the principles perfectly and will naturally follow them as you converse. Take time to discuss each one. Talk with your partner about how each maxim applies to your own case. This will help you both understand that to commit yourselves to a communication partnership is, in effect, to embrace these five principles of effective communication. Clear, caring communication is the ideal to aim for in your communication partnership. Based on the five principles of good communication, clear, caring communication is your mutual commitment to:

- Speaking honestly and clearly.
- Creating an open space where the truth can be said.
- Caring for and supporting one another in your efforts.

Can you do all of this communicating about communication in one conversation? Probably not. Talk with each other about the five principles behind the clear, caring communication as often as necessary to make sure you are fully together in your communication partnership. If you don't get it exactly right at first, be patient with each other and help each other along.

## Communicating about Cupid's Challenge

Once you have committed yourselves to a communication partnership based on clear, caring communication, it's time to put those principles to work. If chronic pain is wreaking havoc on your sex life, it's time to talk about how to deal with that problem.

A main aspect of those discussions will be for you and your partner to work toward understanding just how Cupid's Challenge arises in your relationship. This is, in essence, the *Identify* step of the *ICE* method that we discussed earlier. To identify the problem you need specifics, and you can get a lot of those by asking and answering some key questions such as those related to physiological aspects. But you should also ask questions about other dimensions of the problem. Here are some examples:

How, exactly, is pain affecting your sexual relations? What kind of pain is it? What adjectives best describe it—sharp, achy, burning, tingling? How severe is the pain? During what activities does it occur? What seems to exacerbate the pain? How long does it last? Is it worse on some occasions than on others? What makes the difference? Be specific. Both of you need to understand the details.

Your desires. How do you and your partner each feel about the quality of your sexual relations? What is satisfying about them? What is not so satisfying? Would one or both of you prefer to have sexual relations more often? Less often? What are your specific desires? Are there any new sexual activities that either partner would like to try? Again, be specific.

Your emotions. How do each of you feel about the problem? Overwhelmed? Defeated? Optimistic? Sad? Angry? Identifying your emotions is the first step to being able to deal with them effectively.

Other factors. Are other issues affecting your sex life? Some examples include:

- Are medications having an adverse effect on you or your partner's libido or inhibiting your sexual relations in any other way?
- Are constraints of time or energy impinging on your sex life? Do you tend to have sex so late in the day that one or both partners feel worn out, with little energy left for romance?
- Does the proximity of family members in the home—children, parents, other relatives—make it difficult to find a comfortable time and place for intimacy?
- Are other relationship problems spilling over into the bedroom?

---

Cupid's Point

Can you think of any other factors that might be relevant to the way chronic pain affects a couple's sex lives? In what ways might age play a role for some couples? How about differing libidos or partners' differing views on the purpose and value of sex? Do any of these affect how Cupid's Challenge arises for you and your mate?

---

Once you have a clear understanding of how chronic pain is affecting your sexual relations and what factors are involved, you will be better equipped to determine specific steps for dealing with the issues as referred to in the *Choose* step of *ICE*. As you propose solutions, don't be satisfied with vague statements such as "Well, let's just try to do better." Of course you want to do better, but the best way to do that is to understand the particular problems the two of you are facing and then determine a set of actions to address those problems.

Thus, you need an action plan. This could be as simple as deciding to explore new intercourse positions to reduce strain on one or both partners. Or it might involve a number of elements such as improvements in diet, new sexual activities, changes in the way you communicate in bed, when and where you have sex, or others. It all depends on the specific ways in which Cupid's Challenge arises for you.

You will of course find many ideas in this book to consider as you develop your action plan—ideas on health, attitude, innovative activities, and much more. Locate the ones that are appropriate for your particular case and incorporate them into an action plan that is specifically suited to help the two of you achieve the sexual enjoyment and satisfaction you want and deserve.

Then, as you enact your plan as referred to in the *Explore* step of *ICE,* keep your communication partnership strong. Strive for clear, caring communication as you talk with each other about how well the plan is working. Are the problems being alleviated somewhat, but not enough? What can you do to make the plan even more effective? Keep on communicating, giving each other feedback, and focusing on your goal for a steadily improving sexual relationship.

## More Communication Strategies

We have spent considerable time learning some main principles of good communication and how they fit into a partnership committed to The Three C's. But there are a number of other specific techniques and strategies, some of which are closely related to the foundation we've discussed, that can help you and your partner communicate effectively.

### Understand Your Body Language

You communicate not only with your words and the tone of your voice, but with your eyes, hands, posture, and in fact with your entire body. Remember Mary? She was even communicating something with her headaches: "Not tonight, thank you." Fortunately, with the help of her physician, she was able to recognize the underlying message that her headaches were signaling.

Realize that in your conversations about Cupid's Challenge, your body language can undercut what your words are expressing to your lover. For example, if you want him or her to know that you are fully engaged in the conversation, your message may get garbled if you say it with your eyes closed and your head drooping as if you are falling asleep. Be aware of your partner's body language too. Does it seem to be suggesting something different from what he or she is saying? If so, talk about it in a gentle but honest manner.

In bed, your body speaks especially eloquently because it's your fundamental tool to communicate your desire for and appreciation of your partner. Understand that to convey your excitement, you don't have to be doing somersaults all over your mattress. You can show great desire just by how you look at your partner, or the way you use your hands or lips. Sometimes a caress can veritably shout out what words can not.

## Set Aside a Place and Time to Communicate about Cupid's Challenge

It's a good idea, especially when you first start talking about whatever problems you may be having, to set aside a special time and place to do so. Be sure to give yourselves enough time so that neither of you feels the conversation is rushed. Try to schedule your dialogue for a location and hour where you will have minimal interruption.

In some cases, talking about the issues in bed may be appropriate. If there are others in the household, the bedroom can serve as a conversational refuge where you can have optimum privacy. And if your conversation should turn toward experimentation, or otherwise become erotic, you are in the right place. However, for some couples the bed may be the wrong location for early conversations about Cupid's Challenge. If their sex life has fallen off, or if there are resentments or other relationship matters to be addressed, a more neutral atmosphere may be preferable. Also, try to choose a time for your conversation at which you and your partner are mentally alert. By creating a relaxed atmosphere in which there are few time constraints, you will help make space for truly open communication.

## Don't be Restricted to One Place or Time

Even though it may be important to set aside some special times to talk about Cupid's Challenge, especially when you first start communicating about it, you should be ready to discuss the relevant issues at any time that works for the two of you. For example, if you are reading this book and come across an idea that strikes you as potentially useful, don't feel you need to make an appointment before sharing it with your partner.

Ongoing communication is healthy communication. Your mutual project of improving your sex life while coping with chronic pain should rest on an ongoing dialogue that suits the rhythms of your partnership, which includes both spontaneity and planning. And let's hope those lead to sexy moments in bed!

## Communicate Positively and Avoid Either/Or Stances

In discussing Cupid's Challenge, you will likely need to talk about what is hurtful or what is not working well in your relationship. But you should also try to focus on what does work. What is right about your sexual relations? What feels good? Identify whatever is strong and positive in your relationship and build on that.

Focus on the positive in the way you communicate your thoughts and feelings to your partner. Steer clear of negative labeling, and never deride the other person. Between the two of you, create a positive scenario of how you want things to be, then focus on how to bring that about.

It is also best to avoid either/or stances and instead seek mutual ground on which you two can stand. If your partner wants one thing and you want another, don't think the only solution is that only one of you will get what you want while the other must be disappointed. Keep talking, dig deeper, and try to understand each other better. Seek a solution that will satisfy the deepest needs for both of you.

## Be Big. Both of You

Being "big" means that both partners consider it crucial to understand the other person. Each of you already knows to some extent your own self and how you feel. Now it's time to also understand the issues from your partner's perspective. What does that other person sitting across from you think and feel about your situation? What works best for him or her?

Like good communication itself, being big is a two-way street. If one person reaches out to try to understand the other while the other is interested only in expressing his or her own ideas and feelings and is otherwise oblivious, a serious imbalance in the communication will likely arise. Individual selfishness to the exclusion of the other person has no place in a communication partnership. Any selfishness should be selfishness of the WE. From what each partner thinks and feels individually, the couple should strive to discover what WE want as a couple, what OUR options are, and what WE can and will do to make things better.

If you and your partner find that the all-important WE seems to be missing from your communication, then it's time to review the principles underlying your communication partnership. Start with The Three C's: clear, caring communication. It's about making a space where both partners can be heard and about trying hard to understand each other. It's about being gracious, respectful, engaged, and supportive of one another as you communicate.

In one small word, it's about being "big."

# Chapter Eight

## The Arrow of Appreciation

Of Cupid's many arrows, none can more quickly and dramatically refresh a relationship, even when living with chronic pain, than the Arrow of Appreciation.

This is because one of our most basic human needs is to be thought well of by others. As young children, we hoped to be appreciated by our parents and teachers. Later, it was the regard of our friends that we hungered for, and then the admiration of members of the opposite sex. Now, as adults, there are numerous people we hope will value us for one reason or another: our boss because we are diligent; our co-workers because we are dependable and helpful; our children because we love and sacrifice for them; our neighbors because we are friendly and neighborly.

It is of course important that we validate ourselves as much as possible too. For most of us, though, the person from whom we most desire appreciation is our partner. It is natural to look to our mate for positive answers that typically come in the form of expressions of appreciation. This is largely because it is usually our partner who knows us best and who we feel is best qualified to validate us when we feel vulnerable. Am I a good person? Honest? Reliable? Smart? Attractive? Am I a person worth knowing? Worth loving?

Which brings up a problem—it's become a cliché that partners who have been together for some time often take each other for granted. Over the years, they may have grown used to one another's faces, bodies, and ways of acting and talking. They no longer see in one another the vibrant, fascinating person who once so easily made their body react sexually. Now, to each other, they are like the living room furniture they have had for years—comfortable perhaps, but barely noticed much of the time. No longer are they often struck by what is special about their partner. Seldom do they recall what drew them together in the first place. And as a result, they rarely express their appreciation for one another.

---

Cupid's Point

Take the time to make a list of the main qualities that you see in your partner. For each item on the list, ask yourself when was the last time you complimented him or her on that quality or on doing something that expressed it.

Do you think you express enough appreciation for your partner? Does he or she show enough appreciation for you?

---

Even worse, conflicts, misunderstandings, and unfulfilled expectations may have led one or both members of the couple to feel just the opposite of appreciation for the other. Instead of holding their partner in high regard, they may harbor deep resentments. Instead of expressing how much they value one another, they may devalue each other with their words, or show contempt with their silence. Appreciation may have been replaced by depreciation.

Whether it's due to resentments that have accrued over time, or is simply the result of partners taking each other for granted, countless partnerships are starving for appreciation. These are relationships in which one or both partners want and need—sometimes desperately— recognition, validation, and admiration from the other, but are not getting it. And this lack of appreciation, if it continues, can ravage a couple.

The good news is that the converse is also true, for virtually any relationship can benefit from the Arrow of Appreciation. When partners decide to consistently show their appreciation for one another, they take a big step toward increasing their joy, intimacy, and sexual delight. Mutual appreciation is especially valuable in relationships challenged by chronic pain.

## The Benefits of Appreciation

We have already touched on one main advantage of appreciation—it answers a basic psychological need. We all want to know that we are valuable, and one way we find that out is through feedback from our partner. Getting that feedback can be especially important to individuals dealing with chronic pain because living with such discomfort can leave one mired in self-doubt. Sincere expressions of appreciation help to short circuit negative self-evaluations, reminding these individuals that they are more than just being identified by their pain or condition.

Whereas a lack of appreciation can create a gradually widening chasm in which one or both partners feel that they are not being recognized or respected by the other, or even that they are being taken advantage of or used. Copious expressions of genuine regard do just the opposite. They demonstrate to both partners that they don't take each other for granted and as a result it is natural for such couples to draw closer together. After all, there are few sweeter sounds to hear than words announcing that we are appreciated. We naturally tend to gravitate toward the sources of such words.

Frequent expressions of acknowledgement and thanks also help create a positive mindset about the partnership. It's the epitome of a win-win situation. Partner A expresses appreciation to partner B, and B returns the favor. Back and forth it goes, but not like a closed loop. It's more like a spiral, an upward spiral in which the relationship achieves greater and greater heights as the partners honor and care for each other with true expressions of their regard.

Appreciation can also help us deal more effectively with pain. As we've learned in earlier chapters, and as we may know from experience, having to live with recurring pain often requires sub-stantial psychological and emotional energy. Pain can make us feel weakened, limp, dried up. A dose of appreciation is like a dose of water to the wilted plant. It can momentarily take our minds off our trouble, remind us of who we are, and perk us up. And the more appreciation we get, the perkier we become. Receiving compli-ments and other valuing expressions help us stay psychologically strong, and that's critical if we are to put forth our best efforts to manage our chronic pain wisely and address Cupid's Challenge effectively.

Finally, expressions of appreciation can serve as a wonderful aphrodisiac. Typically, one of the first casualties when one or both partners feel unappreciated by the other is sexual desire. After all, who among us is attracted to someone who doesn't acknowledge us as being valuable? The other side of the coin is that there's little that can make us feel sexier than our partner's sincere demonstrations of appreciation. To feel appreciated is to feel loved and honored for oneself. And there are few things so powerfully seductive as feeling honored by the person we are with.

This seductive effect isn't gender specific. Expressions of appre-ciation work as an aphrodisiac for both women and men. In the bed-room, a woman's sense that she is held in high esteem by her partner tends to make her more receptive to his sexual advances, with this being demonstrated by increased blood flow to her erogenous areas and by the getting-ready-for-you wetness that is a sure mark of desire. A man's sense that he is truly valued by his partner tends to make his blood flow more copiously to his penis and cause seminal fluid to start flowing as his body naturally prepares for sexual activity. In each case, there is a direct connection between being appreciated and the recipient's physiological responses.

## Appreciation Is an Activity

With all of these benefits, you would think that the art of apprecia-tion would be flowering everywhere within partnerships. Yet, many relationships are sadly famished for appreciation. In some cases, however, it's more accurate to say that the relationship is hungry for *expressions* of appreciation. This is because often partners feel quite appreciative of each other, but for some reason they hold back from expressing it. This is the kind of situation that a patient of mine, I'll call him Bill, found himself in.

## Bill and Debbie's Story

*"I know she loves me," Bill said, "but I sometimes feel like the real me is invisible to her." Bill, who had rheumatoid arthritis, was at an evening talk I had been giving about the importance of partners working together when one or both are dealing with chronic pain. Afterward, he had come up to say how much he enjoyed the talk. He told me he agreed with the premise of the presentation and knew that his wife Debbie, who had been unable to attend due to a cold, would have also agreed. She always tried hard to help him deal with his ailment, he said. But it also seemed to him that she never recognized much about him other than his disability.*

*"A lot of the time I feel practically worthless—like I'm nothing more than a burden to her," he said, almost vehemently. "Not that she treats me like a burden. However, she does treat me like an invalid.*

*"But I'm not. I'm not just a guy with arthritis and chronic pain. I hold down a good job—I'm an accountant—and I try to do my part around the house as much as possible. But she doesn't seem to recognize that aspect of me. She gives me lots of sympathy. She always takes my condition into consideration. But she doesn't give me any acknowledgement for the things I do. She never says 'thank you for this' or 'I appreciate you for doing that.' There's never any recognition of me as a full person."*

*I asked him if he had talked to his wife about his feelings.*

*"Not really," he replied. "She does so much for me that I hate to complain to her."*

*"Instead of thinking of it as complaining," I suggested, "you could view it as simply communicating to her something you feel deeply*

*about. If she loves you, don't you think she deserves to understand how you really feel?"*

*"I guess that makes sense," he said, nodding. "I'll think that over."*

*I saw Bill a few weeks later for a checkup and he couldn't wait to tell me that he had taken my suggestion and talked to his wife about his need to feel appreciated by her. "It was a wonderful talk!" he said. "She told me it had never crossed her mind that I would think she didn't appreciate me. Then she proceeded to go through this long list of things that she was grateful to me for—working hard, helping her with the meals and with the kids, bringing her gifts on her birthday, making jokes, my attitude toward life."*

*He went on to say that Debbie had been genuinely surprised when he told her that she never expressed recognition of any of those qualities. She said she had been so appreciative of him in her mind that she was sure she must have often expressed those feelings outwardly. But in the end, she admitted that it was true—her husband's worth was something that she often thought about, but seldom actually told him about.*

*"Now I can't get her to shut up about what a great guy I am," Bill said, laughing. "But the truth is, I love every word of it."*

*"And do you find now that you express your appreciation of her more?" I asked.*

*"Do I? You should hear the two of us. We're the mutual admiration society. Anybody else listening in would probably become jealous. We are thriving on it."*

The important moral here is that true appreciation is an activity, not just a feeling or a thought. It wasn't that Debbie didn't think well of Bill. That wasn't the problem. The problem was the fact that she never showed him how she felt. Not being a mind reader, he concluded that she didn't actually feel much appreciation for him.

For others this oversight can come in the form of a wife or girlfriend being disappointed that her husband or boyfriend never shows his appreciation. When told of this, he is surprised that she feels unappreciated because he actually appreciates her tremendously. It's just that he never gets around to expressing it. But as Bill's story shows, it can work the other way around too. A woman may appreciate her partner yet seldom express it, with the result being that the man feels, understandably, unappreciated by her.

It's important to remember that true appreciation is not something done only in the privacy of our thoughts. If we keep that life-giving nurturance dammed up in our minds, if we never open the spigot of expression, there is no way the gratitude can do its important work.

There are two basic ways we can carry on the activity of appreciation: through our words and our actions.

## Appreciative Words

A usually simple yet very effective way of showing appreciation for our partner is through words. Words of appreciation are mental caresses. Like physical caresses, they show that we value who our partner is. A brief comment such as "You look beautiful tonight" or "Thank you for being so understanding of my mood these days" can be quite powerful and bring a lot of pleasure to our partner.

But here's the mystery: Given that uttering a few words of appreciation is a relatively simple activity, why do so many couples find themselves bereft of such words? Often, even in close relationships in which the partners proclaim they love each other, one or both members of the couple rarely utter a compliment or any other words showing they value their partner.

In some cases, about the only words of appreciation the couple communicates to each other are on greeting cards. But why should we make that extra trip to the store, stand in front of a card rack for fifteen minutes trying to find "just the right card," and end up with one that reads, "I know I never say it, but I think you're the greatest"? Wouldn't it be easier, as well as more personal and effective, to actually say some appreciative things to our partner once in a while?

The dearth of appreciative remarks in a relationship is sometimes due to embarrassment. This seems to happen to men more than to women. Maybe it's because the man was raised in a family in which such comments were seldom made by his father. As a result, appreciative words tend to get jumbled. For him, going fifty miles out of his way to buy a card is preferable to having to come up with one original statement of regard or admiration for his partner.

But it's not just men who can be impoverished when it comes to making appreciative statements. There are also many women who, like Bill's wife Debbie, seldom express such feelings. Some people blame this on a lack of time or energy. After all, for both women and men, life is often a hectic exercise from sunup to late night. So they may find it easy to convince themselves that taking the time to express appreciation for their partner is a chore for which there isn't enough time.

Of course, that's tantamount to believing that to express words showing recognition, respect, and affection to our partner is too much work. If we love our partner though, showing our appreciation will be a pleasure that adds joy to our life, not another chore that we somehow have to fit into our busy schedule.

So let's focus for a moment on two of the simplest and most effective ways of showing our appreciation.

### The Many Reasons to Say "Thank You"
Whatever our reason may be for not expressing appreciative words to our partner—embarrassment, perceived lack of time, forgetfulness, or something else—an excellent way to immediately get into the appreciative spirit is to reacquaint ourselves with two of the most beautiful words in the English language: *Thank you.*

To thank your partner for something is a pure act of appreciation. This is because the words "thank you" accomplish two fundamental things. First, they show you recognize there is something valuable that your partner did, is doing, or will do. Second, they make clear that you think your partner is valuable for doing that thing. It's this second aspect that constitutes the appreciative part. To say "thank you" is tantamount to saying "I value you."

And aren't there always things that we can thank our partner for? Someone once mentioned to me that she would be happy to say "thank you" to her husband if he ever did anything she was thankful for. I expressed my surprise at this. After all, didn't he go to work every day to help support their family? "That's different," she said. "He has to do that."

I pointed out to her that actually he didn't have to do that. Like Gauguin, he could leave his job and family and go to Tahiti to live the life of an artist.

"Fat chance. He can't paint worth a darn," she said, missing my point.

The point was that our partner is probably doing any number of worthwhile things on a regular basis, but because they are repetitive, mundane activities, we may take them for granted and fail to show our appreciation for them. Cooking the meals, washing the dishes, working to make a living, running the kids to their practices, getting the car serviced, painting the hall, cleaning the bathroom—these and countless other everyday jobs are often called "thankless tasks" for good reason; because the person doing the task is seldom thanked.

But why should such actions be taken for granted just because they are done over and over? In fact, isn't that commitment all the more reason to show gratitude?

An excellent way for partners to increase the appreciation they express to each other is to consider all the many ordinary tasks that the other does on a regular or semi-regular basis, and then take the time to offer clear expressions of thanks for their efforts. Even for those who have difficulty finding the right words to express their appreciation, just simply saying "thank you" can go a long way. What could be easier than to give our partner a hug and say, "Honey, I just wanted to thank you for…" and then fill in the rest with whatever fits. And if we put a little thought into it, we probably will find much that does fit; lots of reasons to give lots of kudos.

---

**Cupid's Point**

Make a list of the repetitive tasks that your partner typically does. Include daily tasks like going to work or cooking meals, less frequent tasks like cleaning the oven or mowing the lawn, and still less frequent tasks like doing the taxes, getting the car tuned, or putting on a happy face to visit the in-laws.

Do you thank your partner for doing them? If not, is it because they are expected? Or because they are repetitive? Is either a good reason not to thank your partner for doing them?

Now list the "thankless" tasks that you yourself do repetitively. Does your partner ever thank you for doing any of them?

Ask your partner to do this exercise with you and compare lists. Then talk about what you found out.

---

## Compliments on Appearance

One of the most powerful ways to express appreciation to your partner verbally is to comment favorably on his or her appearance. Below are a few easy examples:

- Your hair always smells so good.
- That shirt looks nice on you.
- I've always loved that dimple.
- You have beautiful eyes.

Who wouldn't respond favorably to hearing such pleasant words? In fact, for most of us words praising our appearance really touch us. Why? Because we identify so closely with our bodies. When our partner compliments some aspect of our appearance, it's as good as saying that you, the very essence of who you are, is attractive.

And we can always find aspects of our partner's appearance to sincerely appreciate even when the passage of years alters their once youthful beauty. Because there is physical beauty at each stage of life if we only have the eyes to see it. If we can't detect the physical beauty in our partner, that tells more about our powers of perception than it does about our partner's physical state. To strive to see, appreciate, and express what we find to be uniquely attractive about our partner is a most rewarding experience, and one that we would do well to cultivate.

Such words can be especially potent if our partner is beset by chronic pain. Because persistent pain is a physical manifestation arising from a bodily ailment or condition, its presence tends to cause those affected by it to feel anything but physically attractive. Words praising some aspect of our partner's appearance can be especially welcome because they contradict that mindset. They assure our partner that he or she remains physically attractive to us.

## Sincerity and Specificity

Whether we are complimenting our partner's appearance, expressing our gratitude, or verbalizing our appreciation in some other way, sincerity is always crucial. There is sometimes a danger of uttering words such as "You look nice tonight" or even "Thank you" while meaning them only halfheartedly when we feel we need to say something appreciative out of a sense of duty. In those instances we may say the first thing that comes to our mind without really thinking about it or even believing it.

To be truly felt by your partner and to have their often wonderful effect, your words of appreciation must express how you really feel. Of course it's necessary for the recipient of those expressions to be receptive to them. You may have met people who simply could not take a compliment, perhaps because they thought poorly of themselves or because they were skeptical of any such statements and dismissed them as insincere. If words or acts of appreciation are to have any benefit, it's crucial to be open to them, especially to sincere expressions that come from your partner.

Specificity is another important aspect of expressing appreciation. Instead of being satisfied with saying something very general such as "I appreciate you" or "Thank you for being you," it's more effective to focus on particular qualities and actions that you can compliment your partner on.

For instance:

- I've been meaning to tell you how much I appreciate you always being in such a good humor.
- You really worked hard raking the leaves today.
- That dress looks nice on you.
- Thanks for running me to the store. I really appreciate that.

To make your words of appreciation specific is to aim the Arrow of Appreciation with precision. By doing so, you demonstrate that you have taken the time to notice some special quality or action belonging to your partner, one that you think is so valuable that it's worth remarking on.

### Appreciative Actions

Expressing your appreciation to your partner through words is a kind of action, but now let's talk about actions that go beyond words. After all, those are usually the most powerful ways to demonstrate appreciation.

For example, it's good when a man or woman often verbally expresses their appreciation for their partner working overtime so they can more quickly save the money for a down payment on a house. Or if she is working late, that extra step he takes in picking up the laundry from the cleaners so she has her favorite pantsuit ready for tomorrow's important business meeting can make a big difference in their love and appreciation for one another. The same is true when she helps him make coffee or breakfast before they both rush out the door to get to work. Or in the case of a stay-at- home mom when he regularly compliments her on how well she runs the house while taking care of the kids.

For couples that still prefer more traditional male and female roles, he can show his appreciation by occasionally breaking free from that traditionalism and rising up from the dinner table to clear the plates, put away the food, and wash the dishes, allowing her to retire to the family room to relax half an hour earlier than she would otherwise be able to; and she can occasionally equally chip in with the "honey-do list" usually set aside for him.

The reason appreciative actions speak so powerfully to your partner, regardless of the nature of your relationship, is that they require extra effort. No wonder appreciative actions tend to mean so much.

## Cherish Lists

Of course, an action meant to be appreciative serves that purpose well only if it provides something that your partner truly wants. Otherwise, it may backfire. The man who gives his partner a new vacuum cleaner for her birthday to show his appreciation for how well she keeps up the house may be doing exactly right by her if she has been complaining about her old vacuum cleaner and strongly signaling that she would like a new one. But if she has been hinting that what she would like is a watch that she saw at the jewelry store, she may consider the vacuum cleaner gift to be evidence not of her partner's appreciation, but of his obliviousness to what would truly please her. The same could be said if she gives him a hedge trimmer when he's been talking about wanting tickets to go see his favorite sports team play the next time they're in town.

Knowing your partner's Cherish List is a good way to avoid this problem. A Cherish List is a list of a few things we hold dear to our hearts and that we would like to receive from our partner. This may include special gifts or activities, but it may also include relatively mundane items that have special importance to the recipient. By giving us something on our Cherish List, our partner shows us that we are cherished and treasured.

We all have such a list, and that certainly includes those of us who live with persistent pain. In fact, some of the elements on our list may directly arise from the challenge that chronic pain presents to us. One woman who was living with severe joint pain had the following Cherish List, which included several items that reflected the fact that she often felt housebound:

- For my husband to show he cherishes me by taking me on a Sunday drive in the country.
- For the two of us to have a night out once a month, and for it to be a planned night out so that we can have the pleasure of anticipation.
- For my husband to give me flowers, or even just a single rose, on my birthday and Valentine's Day and sometimes on just an ordinary day to show that he is thinking of me.
- For my husband to have one day each week when he takes over the cooking and after-dinner chores freeing me up for a "dinner-holiday."

When Cherish Lists stay private or are barely spoken of, it can be difficult for our partner to understand which actions or other gifts we would hold most dear. Sometimes even we ourselves don't understand what's most important to us and need to take the time to come up with our Cherish List before we can tell our partner.

An especially synergistic way to communicate about Cherish Lists is for both members of the couple to make up their own lists and share them with one another. Making it into a joint activity counteracts any thought that either partner is being selfish in sharing his or her special desires.

Cupid's Point

List the things that your partner could give you or do for you that would make you feel most cherished. Yes, I know you want a Ferrari or a three-carat diamond pendant! But list only things and actions that are currently within your partner's range and that you would regard as true signs of cherishing you.

If you are living with chronic pain, are any of the items on the list associated with that reality?

Then look at his or her Cherish List. Do any of the things on the list surprise you? How well do you think you would do in fulfilling their requests?

## Going on an Appreciation Date

At this point, you may be thinking that all of this talk about appreciation sounds well and good, but to get your partner to express appreciation verbally or otherwise is a task much easier said than done.

This is certainly true for some relationships, whether the partners are dealing with chronic pain or not. And of course appreciation is most rewarding when mutually expressed and not just a one-way street. This then offers an opportunity for you and your partner to engage together in your understanding of appreciation so the two of you will be on the same page.

In other relationships though, one partner, or both, may remain relatively oblivious to the importance of appreciation. Or even if both realize its importance, the hubbub of everyday life may lead them to forget. It helps if the couple can find a way to focus their attention on the topic of appreciation so they can clearly acknowledge to themselves and each other its importance to their relationship.

One way to do this is to go on an appreciation date. This is just what its name implies. It's a special time set aside for the purpose of focusing on and developing a more appreciative relationship. An appreciation date can include an evening out to dinner or to some romantic hideaway, or the partners may decide to stay home. In either case, it is ideal to make their date into a special event, one with a relaxed atmosphere and plenty of time to talk.

If an appreciation date seems like a good idea for you and your partner, one way to approach it is to divide it into three main parts:

Appreciating your history together. You begin your date by talking about and celebrating your history as a couple—how you met, your courtship, your early years, and on to the present. What times of your lives together do you remember with most pleasure? What are your favorite specific recollections? To help refresh your memory, you may want to enjoy some of your photographs from past years. Going over your history together can help you recall and articulate what is good about your relationship. It reminds you of where you have been, of who you are together, and of what you want to achieve as a couple. Whether you do it at home over a shared bowl of popcorn, or at a restaurant as you enjoy a nice meal, this can make for a most delightful conversation.

Appreciating each other. Talking about what is valuable about your relationship will naturally lead to expressing your appreciation for one another. This is the second main part of your appreciation date. To begin, one partner expresses something that he or she likes about the other, then the other returns the favor. This may go back and forth through a second bowl of popcorn, or a lingering dessert, or even further. The idea is for you both to express from the heart what it is you like and admire about each other.

Committing to appreciation. The third main part of your appreciation date is to commit yourselves to making *appreciation* an integral part of your lives. This may be an easy commitment to make because you will have been experiencing the power of appreciation and the closeness it generates.

I think many of the women reading this will fall in love with the idea of an appreciation date, but for some of you men out there who may not be convinced of its value, I hope you'll give it your very best try anyway. Following through may seem a bit awkward at first, but it may be easier than you think once you begin talking about the good memories you have of your relationship and what you love and appreciate about your partner. Realize that an appreciation date is simply a celebration of each other and your relationship. Give it a chance, and it's likely to pay off not only in a nice evening together with your special lady, but very possibly in the bedroom for many nights to come.

In fact, a periodic appreciation date can be a good way to renew your relationship on a continuing basis. Your history together is likely to be so rich that there will be more good memories to be recalled in subsequent dates and more qualities for you and your partner to identify with and celebrate.

## Appreciation in the Bedroom

Mutual appreciation should have an honored place in any bedroom, and certainly when chronic pain is an issue. The many advantages of appreciation joined together in the bedroom help create an atmosphere in which couples can deal most effectively with Cupid's Challenge. Some examples include:

A sexy atmosphere. Expressions of appreciation create a sexier, more seductive atmosphere in the bedroom. While pain has a way of making us feel less than physically perfect, complimentary words tend to counteract the discomfort. If we are afflicted by pain, appreciative words can assure us of our continued sexual attractiveness, which is a big part of feeling sexy.

A positive atmosphere. Feeling appreciated also helps both partners, particularly the one dealing directly with the pain, to maintain a positive, empowering attitude in the bedroom. The feedback from our partner showing us that we are valued greatly contributes to positivity.

An intimate atmosphere. We know that mutual expressions of appreciation tend to draw couples closer together. In the bedroom, this results in an atmosphere of intimacy. Generally, the most pleasurable sex is emotionally intimate and mutual appreciation is perfectly designed to enhance such closeness.

A relaxed atmosphere. Complimenting, applauding, cherishing, and otherwise appreciating each other in the bedroom help partners keep the mood light and erotic. Remember Karl and Melissa in chapter six? A few sincere appreciative comments could have helped them lessen the heaviness in their bedroom, relax them both, and enable them to turn a difficult situation into one that was hopeful and sexy.

Overall, mutual expressions of appreciation in the bedroom can be one of the most purely pleasurable and seductive aspects of intimacy thus setting the stage on which Cupid flourishes. It creates an environment that helps both partners realize the other values them, and this in turn tends to generate sexual anticipation and excitement. Also, by focusing on one another, partners are able to lose themselves more completely in the sensuality of the moment.

Yet, couples typically fall into habitual patterns in the way they have sex, and if expressions of appreciation were not a main part of the pattern to begin with, it may never occur to them to give appreciation a bigger role in their sex lives. But when chronic pain enters the picture, former habits may no longer work well and thereby require the partners to discover new ways of enjoying being together. If this describes you and your mate, then one of the very best new habits for you to develop is the art of mutual appreciation.

In the bedroom, this begins with understanding each other. In particular, being aware of your biological rhythms—different individuals may be most amenable to sexual activity at certain times of the day. One may be more aroused early in the morning, another late at night. Understanding your partner's and your own sexual rhythms can be a big step toward understanding how the two of you best fit together.

Achieving a healthy environment of mutual appreciation in the bedroom may require some effort. It will take clear, caring communication and a strong commitment to making appreciation an integral part of your relationship inside and outside of the bedroom. However, that work can quickly prove its worth by fostering a great atmosphere in which your sexual happiness prospers. And that, too, is certainly something to appreciate.

# Chapter Nine

# The Arrow of Touch

While our other faculties are located in our head, touch is situated over the entire surface of our body. Though we have only two eyes, two ears, one nose, and one tongue, our sense of touch encompasses millions of receptors embedded in our skin, from the top of our head to the tips of our toes.

For the most part, these receptors are incredibly sensitive. To see what I mean, have your partner or a friend barely touch, with one finger, the end of a single hair on your head. Or touch it yourself with a small piece of paper. Can you feel how only a slight contact creates a distinct tactile experience on your scalp just below the strand of hair? By bringing us countless such messages—of pressure, vibration, heat, cold, and pleasure—from all over our body's surface, touch enriches us with sensation.

The sum of all those messages helps define us as physical beings. At the same time, they inform us instantly about what we are in contact with at each point of our skin—whether it's rough or silky, wet or dry, hard or soft. And it does so in an especially intimate way because, unlike vision, hearing, and smell, our tactile sense requires actual physical contact with objects. Touch is always up-close and personal.

Maybe that's one reason why touch is so intimately related to our emotions, a truism abundantly reflected in our language. For instance, we use the word *feel* to refer both to making tactile contact with something and to having an emotional experience—*I feel happy, or anxious, or on top of the world.* We also say that something *touched* us when it made a powerful emotional impression on us.

With all of this immediacy, closeness, and emotion built into the sensation of touch, it's no wonder that sex and sensual pleasure are about touch more than any other single sense. Our other faculties are certainly important for sensuality, but our primary sensory organ for erotic delight is our skin with its sense of touch. And after all, scintillating sex is very pleasurable bodily sensations intermixed with strong emotions of desire and affection. Add the fact that the truest ways to physical intimacy are via the pathways of touch, and it's even clearer why our tactile sense forms one half of a very basic equation: Erotic Touch = Sensuality and Pleasure.

This equation is the first of two key aspects of touch that make it so important for couples facing Cupid's Challenge. The second aspect is that all kinds of loving touches, both sensual and nonsensual, serve to bind partners closer together. So let's focus on these two central aspects of touch—bonding and sensuality. When you and your partner put these elements together, touch becomes a wonderful medium through which to address Cupid's Challenge.

## How Pain Complicates Sensual Touch

Let's begin by identifying some main ways that chronic pain can interfere with touch, especially erotic touch. As true as the above equation may be in general, the mathematics of sensual touch are often not so simple for individuals who live with chronic pain. When pain is added to the left side of the equation, the formula can become imbalanced with the right side diminishing or even disappearing altogether.

This can happen in any number of basic ways. In one case, stimulation of an area of our skin that would normally bring us pleasure instead causes pain. This may happen, for example, with reflex sympathetic dystrophy (also known as RSD or as Complex Regional Syndrome I or II), a condition that involves a decreased threshold of pain over one or more areas of the body so that otherwise inoffensive stimuli such as a simple touch can be hurtful.

A second and perhaps more frequent way that pain interferes with sensual touch includes cases in which the pain originates from deeper inside the body; for instance with muscle, joint, and low back pain. Here, the experience of pain tends to diminish or even overwhelm any pleasurable sensations that we might get from sensual touch.

A third way that pain frustrates erotic touch is by interacting with our psychology to diminish sensory pleasure. This kind of circumstance can be illustrated by the plight of Jennifer and Gary with their concerns about pain as it relates to sensual touch.

### Jennifer and Gary's Story

*Jennifer laid in bed trying to hold back her tears. Gary, her husband, had just tried to interest her in making love, but she had rebuffed him again as she had done several times over the last few months. It wasn't that Gary was insensitive in his approach, actually his caresses were gentle. It was just that she knew his touch, if it were to continue, would eventually lead to intercourse and she dreaded the pain that intercourse would bring to her arthritic hip.*

*She had not told Gary what was troubling her because she felt embarrassed at what she considered to be her weakness, ashamed at letting the expectation of pain keep her from gladly receiving her husband's advances. She had only said, "I'm sorry, I'm just tired tonight."*

*Hearing that, Gary had turned over with a sigh.*

*Now, as Jennifer laid there, she told herself that she had been right to stop Gary when she did. She decided that allowing him to continue and then asking him to stop later when the arthritis began acting up would have amounted to leading him on. But telling herself these things didn't much help in relieving her despair.*

*She thought about how close and rewarding their sex life had once been. There had been so many times when Gary's erotic caresses had been welcome, pleasurable, exciting. But recently, their sensual aspect had entirely disappeared. These days, even his slightest touch set off an alarm of anxiety so loud it drowned out any possible plea-sure it might have given her.*

*What was worse was that Gary's attempts to interest her were becoming more and more infrequent. Soon, she feared, his efforts would completely stop.*

*She lifted a tissue out of the box on the bedside table.* It's no good to long for the way things used to be, *she thought as she dried her tears. She set the used tissue on the table, then turned over carefully, so as not to aggravate her hip. Sleep. That's the only thing that made any sense. Just sleep.*

For Jennifer and Gary, the basic Touch-Sensuality-Pleasure equation is badly out of balance. Their situation reveals one of the common ways that pain can keep us from responding to a lover's touch. This is the circumstance where being touched is not painful in itself, but rather it leads to an expectation that pain will eventually arrive if the touching continues. For Jennifer, that expectation raises her anxiety level so high that it negates any pleasure she might receive from her husband's caresses. In fact, it makes her positively want him not to touch her.

The clear advice for Jennifer and Gary is for them to embark on the *ICE* strategy by identifying and communicating about their problem in bed. Jennifer needs to tell her husband what she is thinking and feeling so he will understand the role pain is playing in her refusals. Once that's done, they can start figuring out how to deal with it. Taking whatever advice and relief Jennifer's physician may be able to offer, the couple can choose and then begin exploring methods to address the problem—including ways to restore touch to its proper place in their relationship.

That's the fun part. But to go about it effectively, the couple needs a solid understanding of touch and how to use it. That's crucial, because their apparent lack of sensual savvy about touch seems to be part of their problem. In particular, they need to understand the two key aspects of touch—sensuality and bonding.

## The Importance of Nonsexual Bonding Touch

If we want to use touch to enhance our sexual pleasure even when dealing with chronic pain, there's probably no better place to start than by realizing the inestimable value of nonsexual touch. If this seems like a paradox, just consider for a moment the many ways we have of affectionately touching our partners—caressing, cuddling, embracing, fondling, kissing, hand-holding, licking, pecking, patting, rubbing, shoulder-touching, stroking, and more—each with its own meaning and message.

Some of these ways, such as petting, typically have a pronounced sexual connotation. Others, such as hugging and hand-holding, often have no sexual overtones. But that certainly doesn't mean they aren't important for a couple's sexual togetherness, for if nonsexual ways of touching are rare or missing in a partnership, the sexual side of the relationship is probably misdirected too.

This is because affectionate nonsexual touching is a fundamental way for partners to bond. In fact, such touches are so important for the process of joining couples that we can call them *bonding touches*. Of course, sexual touches usually serve to bond partners together too and often are referred to as *sensual* and *erotic touches*.

Bonding touches can express volumes of meaning. For one thing, they signify our acknowledgment and acceptance of our partner. With a simple hug, a holding of hands, a little nudge in jest as we stroll with our loved one, we are saying to him or her, "I love you just as you are."

And what an important message that is! All of us experience times when the world seems against us, when we feel that people don't accept us for ourselves. On such occasions, our partner's expression of unconditional acceptance through a timely touch can be a priceless gift. In fact, kisses on the cheek, affectionate embraces, and other bonding touches are among the most important bits of glue cementing our partnerships.

The fact that bonding touches serve this purpose is no surprise. It's a lesson we all learned very early when we were infants and the loving touches of our mother and father communicated a message of acceptance and acknowledgement. Now, as adults, we pass that lesson along to our own children. What is the first thing we do when we rise in the middle of the night to tend to a crying baby? We touch the child to reassure him or her that mommy or daddy is there because we know instinctively that our gentle but firm touch will relay a message of comfort, acknowledgement, acceptance, support, and security.

Using bonding touches to show acceptance and support can be especially important if our partner lives with the challenge of chronic pain. And as we know, living with chronic pain day after day can result in negative emotions and thoughts. Indeed, chronic pain survivors sometimes feel that their condition makes them somehow inadequate in comparison to others. They may have a sense of guilt about their situation, or they may feel they are a burden to others. Expressing our acceptance of our partner through bonding touches can be a powerful antidote for such self-harming thought patterns.

In addition, affectionate nonsexual touches can have a physiologically beneficial effect. They tend to lower blood pressure, relieve emotional stress, and release endorphins, creating pleasurable feelings that can help counteract pain.

Not only do bonding touches signal our acceptance and support, they also serve as deep signifiers of our love. Such simple touches can eloquently express that we cherish the other person and signal our devotion. Yet ironically, by carrying such a strong message of love, nonsexual touches can act as a powerful aphrodisiac.

This is something that many people don't understand well. It can be difficult for a woman, as well as for a man, to be truly desirous of sexual activity and to respond positively to her partner's advances if she doesn't believe that he truly loves her. One of the main ways she makes this judgement is by how and how often her partner touches her in nonsexual contexts. Does he ever embrace her for no reason other than to show her he loves her? Does he sometimes come up behind her as she relaxes in a chair after a long day and massage her shoulders, showing her that he recognizes she works hard? So if her partner seldom expresses his affection through embraces, kisses, or other affectionate nonsexual touches, she may conclude that he has little genuine regard for her.

Unfortunately, even in these better-informed times, some men are still brought up with the idea that touching is somehow unmanly unless it's sexually motivated. If a man's parents, and perhaps especially his father, did not show him much affection through touch when he was a child, or if he seldom observed his father affectionately touching his mother, he may be living out that misguided lesson in his adult life. There is nothing unmanly about affectionate nonsexual touching, whether it's hugging your partner, kissing your child, or patting your buddy on his back.

While hesitancy to engage in bonding touch may reflect a man's upbringing, it doesn't necessarily indicate his actual feelings for his partner. This was brought out especially well in the case of one couple, Jason and Lynn. Jason often gave his wife, Lynn, gifts on special occasions and even sometimes on a garden-variety Tuesday, and he usually included a nice card that expressed his affection for her.

But Jason seldom touched Lynn in an affectionate, nonsexual way. Even when they had sex, he never held her afterward, and only rarely did he embrace her or venture to hold her hand outside of bed. As a result, Lynn started believing that he didn't really love her. She suspected that the cards and gifts were a ploy to fool her into thinking that he cared for her.

It wasn't until their marriage hit some sizable bumps that Jason discovered how his wife felt. At a counseling session, he was flabbergasted to learn that she suspected him of not loving her.

"But I love you very much," he protested.

"You never show it," she replied.

"Not true! I bring you gifts all the time!"

"But they're not the ones I need. You never hug me, never just hold me. Those are the gifts I want the most!"

As he listened to her, Jason began understanding that the most meaningful way to express his love for Lynn—most meaningful to *her*—was to touch her in ways that directly and immediately expressed his loving feelings. That day he learned something important about her Cherish List, and when he began acting on that knowledge, most of the marital bumps faded away. And yes, he even continued bringing her cards and gifts.

Too often, one or both members of a couple don't realize the importance of nonsexual bonding touch. If we return to Jennifer and Gary for a moment, we can see that it's especially important for them, given their situation, to understand the power of nonsexual touch. This is because Gary's caresses in bed have come to trigger anxiety in Jennifer's mind, and there's some danger that all of his touches, sexual or nonsexual, might start evoking her anxious thoughts.

One approach this couple can work on is to give each other plenty of hugs and other bonding touches, where it's understood that nothing sexual is implied or expected. And that the touching is just a way to show their love and affection for each other.

The same goes for virtually all of us. When a couple is having sexual difficulties, it's beneficial for them to engage in more bonding touch. By doing so, they assure each other that despite their current problems in bed, they still love and support one another. By cuddling, holding hands, and otherwise displaying their affection through nonerotic touch, they are saying to each other, "I love you. And we'll work through this thing together."

So far we've mostly talked about what affectionate, nonsexual touches mean for the recipient—that he or she is acknowledged, accepted, reassured, supported, loved, and cherished. But they are also meaningful to the giver. To be able to express our affection for the one we love through touching is, for most of us, a necessity. It's almost impossible to love someone without wanting to express those feelings, and for the majority of us, a very natural way to do that is through embraces and other bonding touches.

---

Cupid's Point

A great time to express your feelings through bonding touches can be while you and your partner are talking about how chronic pain is affecting your relationship. Such conversations can be difficult due to embarrassment or feelings of guilt.

How might you and your mate use bonding touch to reduce anxiety as you discuss how Cupid's Challenge is affecting your lives? For example, holding hands while you talk.

Bonding touches help ease a conversation by showing your love for and acceptance of each other. They can also signify that you are going to work together to face the challenge of chronic pain as a loving and sexual team.

---

This is important for those of us living with chronic pain to remember—that to be active givers of touch is as important to our wellbeing as being welcoming receivers. Don't allow your chronic pain to make you be only a recipient of this beautiful form of communication. But rather look for comfortable ways to reciprocally reach out to and actively express your love and affection for your partner through touch.

## The Second Main Aspect: Erotic Touch as an Appetizer and an End in Itself

Erotic touch is fundamental to sexual pleasure. However, it is thoroughly underappreciated by millions of men and women in our society. Instead of giving it high honor, many couples treat it merely as a means to an end. This approach to sensual touch can often be traced to a misplaced "macho" attitude. Some men may view it as being little more than a set of requirements to be met, a series of procedures that he must go through in order to get his partner "hot" enough so they can progress to the "big event," intercourse.

But it's not always just the man who is responsible for this way of viewing sensual touch. The female as half of the partnership sometimes falls right into step with the idea. She never realizes that there can be much more to erotic touch than a few hurried caresses motivated by a desire to quickly arrive at the climax.

It is important to note though that if viewing sexual touch solely as a quick means to an end works well for both members of a couple, then more power to them. However by taking such a restricted view of erotic touch, they are greatly limiting their possibilities for sexual enjoyment. And for many couples, employing sensual touch only as a means to an end may work well for a time, but eventually it more often can lead to conflict and heartache.

This may be especially true for couples dealing with chronic pain. As an illustration, consider again Jennifer and Gary's situation where there's evidence that an attenuated view of sensual touch is part of their problem. As gentle as Gary's caresses may be, he seems to be using them mainly as a way to prepare Jennifer for the idea of intercourse. If so, his plan isn't working. In fact, Jennifer's perception that his caresses must eventually lead to intercourse is causing her to tell him to stop. Gary's caresses aren't actually erotic for Jennifer. She experiences them only as signifying eventual pain.

The irony here is that what is working against the couple, sensual touch, is the very thing that could help them achieve a more satisfying sexual relationship. For that to happen, it's important for Jennifer and Gary to develop a better understanding and a deeper appreciation of sensual touch. The same is true for many others living with chronic pain. So instead of taking a utilitarian view of erotic touch, you can open up its power to please by treating it as an appetizer, an end in itself, or both.

## Erotic Touch as an Appetizer

To regard sensual touch as an appetizer is to see it as being similar to a plate of tasty, tempting hors d'oeuvres that we enjoy at the beginning of a good meal. Though the appetizer can be considered a lead-in to the main course, it functions as much more if we don't gobble it down too quickly. It is something that we can savor, enjoy, and linger over. That way, the appetizer becomes an integral part of the entire sensual experience of the meal. At the same time, whetting our appetite makes the main course more enjoyable than it would have been otherwise.

You can take the same attitude toward sensual touch. Within a particular encounter, you and your partner may still consider erotic touch as part of a larger process that leads to intercourse. But you can also recognize it as providing its own special pleasures. When you do so, erotic touch becomes caresses to take your time with and delight in. No longer just a means to an end, sensual touch becomes a pleasurable and intrinsic part of the entire delicious sexual encounter. In fact, the longer you linger in the world of erotic touch, the more you may increase your appetite for further sexual activity with your partner.

## Erotic Touch as an End in Itself
You can go even further in your celebration of sensual touch. There's nothing to prevent you and your partner from deciding, on various or perhaps many occasions, to dispense with the idea that your touching is supposed to lead to something else. Instead, you may treat it as being so pleasurable that it becomes its own purpose. Approaching erotic touch from this perspective means understanding that intercourse does not need to be the object of *every* sexual encounter. It means recognizing that partners may gain great pleasure, intimacy, and satisfaction simply from touching each other sensually.

Learning how to approach sensual touch as an end in itself can be especially valuable for couples facing the challenge of chronic pain. That's because focusing on and enjoying touch for its own sake often requires fewer bodily movements and places less stress on muscles and joints than does intercourse. As a result, there may be less chance that pain will interfere with the pleasure of your sexual encounters. With the expectation of pain eliminated, a sexual engagement can unfold in easy, undemanding ways that emphasize sensuous relaxation and luxurious pleasure.

Such encounters may or may not involve orgasm for one or both partners. Either way, they can be satisfying experiences that tap into hidden stores of sensuality. They can also be emotionally fulfilling as the mutual appreciation and pleasuring of one another's body can arouse strong passions and deep feelings of love and togetherness.

## How to Become Better Touchers and Touchees

If erotic touch has played only a cursory role in a couple's lovemaking, they may be unsure of how to make it a fuller part of their relationship. They may feel their skill level isn't high enough and think it awkward to engage in more erotic touching than usual. If you or your partner have such qualms, it's natural for you to wonder how to begin your explorations. Just what steps can you take to become better touchers and touchees?

The quick answer is the same as it would be for most other activities: the best way to learn how to do something new is to just do it. Guidance from books, articles, or a physician may help, but it's only when you discover what works for the two of you in your unique situation that you can really start learning how to best use sensual touch to enhance your sexual relationship.

One often-ignored method to learn about your pleasure zones is to use self-touch. Some women may attach a stigma to masturbation or any other kind of erotic self-touching. As for men, the great majority probably have few qualms about masturbation, but many are hesitant to explore their self-touching sensuality beyond masturbation. In both cases the reluctance is unfortunate, because self-touch can be an excellent resource for discovering how our bodies work. The more we discover what we like through sensual self-exploration, the more clearly we are able to communicate to our partner what pleases us most.

Another way to learn about your sensual self is to undertake an erotic voyage of discovery with your partner. If done with love, patience, and understanding, this journey can be one of your most delightful ways of sharing your love. This voyage of discovery is the perfect time to recall the *ICE* method. First, *Identify* sensual touch as something that you want to make a bigger part of your sexual lives.

Next, discuss your options and *Choose* how to carry out your explorations. Then, *Explore* sensual touch.

In regards to *Choose* and *Explore,* it's important for the two of you to be in agreement about three main aspects of your voyage. These are:

- Your goals for the exploration.
- The atmosphere you want to create.
- How to proceed.

Let's spend some time with each of these aspects, identifying specific ideas as we go along.

## Setting Goals for Exploring Erotic Touch

To maximize the value of your explorations, it's vital to set clear goals and commit yourselves to fulfilling them. Your main goal in sensual exploration is the sharing and enjoyment of each other's company.

Within that context of enjoyment, your secondary goal can be to learn the most pleasurable ways of sensually touching each other. This means learning what one another's erogenous zones are and the most pleasurable ways of stimulating those areas. These are areas of the body that tend to provide the most intense sensual pleasure when touched appropriately. Some people will have less sensitivity to sensual stimulation of their "traditional" erogenous zones than others, and capacities for pleasure will vary.

It's important to realize that many parts of the body that we might not at first think of as erogenous zones could be potential pleasure spots, depending on the person. For instance, some men are receptive to a sensual touch on their nipples, while others find it nonerotic. Many women greatly enjoy having the soles of their feet massaged, whereas others find that to be too ticklish for enjoyment. Virtually any part of the body—stomach, ears, neck, thighs, wrists, even elbows and knees—might serve as an erogenous zone for one individual or another.

Because of these variations, be sure that you and your partner don't assume what each other's pleasure zones are before you have definitive proof. And the proof is in each partner's reactions to sensual touch. That's why *exploration* is essential.

Part of learning about your partner's pleasure zones is to discover the particular ways that he or she prefers to be touched at each pleasure point. A sensual touch may be as light and airy as a hummingbird's feather, or firm and focused. One woman may love her nipples being rolled firmly between her partner's fingers, while another may like them to be brushed with only the most delicate touch. It's also important to remember that what pleases someone may be rather complex at times. For example, a man may respond most fully to his penis being touched lightly at first, and then being grasped more firmly. Or he may prefer to feel one hand barely touching the end of his penis while the other grasps the shaft.

Though discovering how each other likes to be touched is one of the main objectives on your journey, don't let it become a job or a chore. Keep it light, playful, and erotic. Remember, the most important objective of your session is to enjoy your time together. The sense that the both of you are on a delicious adventure, a pleasure cruise into somewhat uncharted but ultimately very warm and friendly waters, can thus permeate your interactions. The secondary aim, to learn about each other's pleasure zones, will tend to fall right into place if you have fun on your adventure.

But what if it turns out that you or your mate don't experience much erotic pleasure from your explorations? If that happens, don't let it spoil the mood. Cuddle, reaffirm your love for one another, talk to each other about what you've learned, and go from there.

## Setting the Atmosphere

There are other specific steps you can take to ensure that your surroundings and attitude are conducive to maximum enjoyment:

Make a firm touch date. Setting a specific date and time to explore sensual touch with one another is crucial to making it happen. Your touch date might comprise anything from an overnight stay in a nice hotel, to retiring early one evening for a special encounter in your own bed. Whatever venue you choose, set aside enough time to conduct your sensual investigations without feeling rushed. Also, try to make arrangements so you won't be interrupted. For instance, turn off the cell phone if possible, ask the grandparents if they can watch the kids for the evening, and make sure the dog has been walked.

Comfort is crucial. Take special care to prepare the physical surroundings such as the bed, pillows, cushions, and room temperature to allow for optimum comfort and reasonable mobility for the partner with chronic pain. Ensure that pain levels are acceptable, meaning not so high as to override the pleasure that may come from sensual touch. Also, a warm bath beforehand may help to relax muscles, loosen joints, and establish the right frame of mind. In the event that pain becomes too great during the session, stop the exploratory activities and set another date to resume.

Create a romantic setting. Candles, soft music, special perfume, or flowers can add even more to the sensuality of your romantic atmosphere.

Be awake and be there. For your erotic touch date, it's important to set aside a time when both of you will be awake, energized, and relaxed. Not ten o'clock on a weeknight, for example, if that's your normal bedtime and you usually fall right to sleep. If you are taking medications that tend to increase tiredness or negatively affect your libido, your physician may be able to prescribe substitute medications with fewer such effects, or perhaps authorize a brief "pharmacological holiday."

It's also important for both of you to be fully present mentally by not letting extraneous thoughts and concerns intrude on your explorations. Do your best to set the worries of the day aside, still the mental chatter, and relax. Don't forget, all you need to "accomplish" on your date is to enjoy your time together.

Be honest and open. The point of exploring sensual touch is not for one partner to try to please the other by saying what he or she thinks the other wants to hear. It's to communicate honestly with each other about what feels good and what doesn't. By doing so, your explorations can serve to make erotic touch a fuller and more enjoyable part of your relationship. Without honesty though, the point is lost.

The other side of being honest is to be open to what the other person truly feels. This means setting aside preconceived ideas about what the other will find pleasurable, and especially about what he or she *should* find pleasurable. True exploration requires an open mind.

Create a safe place. It's crucial for you and your lover to create a safe emotional place for one another during your explorations. Most of us are self-conscious about our body, and exposing ourselves to sensual touch can heighten our sense of vulnerability. It takes trust to reveal oneself truly and fully. Strive, through patience and clear, caring words of love and encouragement to show one another that your trust is well-placed.

---

Cupid's Point

In creating a safe space for each other, be mindful that:

- We all feel self-conscious about our body, so you and your partner may both feel vulnerable in presenting yourselves to each other for sensual touch.
- The partner living with chronic pain may feel especially vulnerable.
- Sweet words of appreciation for your lover and their body can help defuse anxieties. Such words are often highly pleasurable in themselves and can help open the gates to greater erotic pleasure.
- Appreciation can be one of your most valuable assets for making your touch date a great success.

---

## The Exploration

Once you have chosen the right time and place for your erotic touch date and know how to create the right atmosphere, you're almost ready to begin. First though, it's a good idea to create and agree on a plan about how to actually conduct your explorations.

Having a plan can help ensure that initially you will both have an approximately equal amount of time as givers and receivers. But don't feel bound too tightly by your plan. If after your first explorations the heat of the moment results in a mutual decision to throw out the plan and just do what feels good to both of you, that may be one of the best results you could hope for. If that happens, you can set another date on which to continue your more methodical sensual explorations.

Your plan may also include how you will initially proceed in touching each other. For example, you might decide to start with one partner lying on his or her stomach, while the other moves down the recipient's body from head to toe with sensual caresses and kisses— always being especially careful not to irritate any painful or injured area. Then the touchee might turn over to allow the toucher to continue, or the recipient could become the toucher.

A good plan will be somewhat detailed. It will create a structure that enables each partner to know what is supposed to be happening at each step. But don't set it in stone, or it may defeat the idea of exploration. For instance, when the recipient says that something feels especially good, then that's probably the time for the toucher to linger there and explore the area.

Clear communication is important to the success of your explorations. The touchee's body movements and sighs while being touched can be important guides to the toucher, while verbal communication can be quite precise. The toucher may ask questions such as "How does this feel?" or "Which feels better, this or that?" The recipient's replies can help guide their partner's hands. Brief directions such as "Yes, that's nice" or "A little more pressure please" can provide important feedback. Keeping your voices low as you communicate can help you stay in the sexy mood of the moment. Many couples find this kind of back and forth communication about what they are doing with one another to be very erotic in itself.

It's important for you and your mate to learn not only what pleases each other, but also what may be painful or uncomfortable. The toucher should take great care when his or her hands are approaching a locus of pain. If discomfort arises from a touch, the recipient should gently say so. Usually, this can be done clearly and calmly, avoiding alarming responses such as "Don't do that!" and instead "Sweetheart, here would be much better" while guiding the partner's hand to a different, more pleasurable area. This enables the recipient to continue emphasizing the pleasure points and verbalizing pleasure.

On your erotic touch date, you do not have to restrict yourselves to pathways of touch that you have always used before unless there is some sound medical reason. The idea is to explore. It's to try new, creative ways of touching, while always maintaining physical safety and avoiding discomfort.

Realize that sensual touch is mostly a dynamic, not static faculty. As a result, the power of erotic touch to please will typically vary on several dimensions, including the area touched, rhythm, and pressure. As you explore, seek to discover the right combinations that will create the most intense feelings of erotic pleasure in each other.

---

Cupid's Point

Gentle, sensual touch of an area that is normally a point of pain can sometimes be a pleasing part of the exploratory process. This kind of touch may be soothing both physically and emotionally. Maybe that's because it evokes feelings similar to those experienced in childhood when a parent gently touched a scraped elbow and soothed hurt feelings.

Realize that comforting words can be a most important part of such an exploration. If you are the recipient, what words and tone would you want to hear from your partner as you are being touched? If you are the giver, what do you think your mate would want to hear? Do this exercise together and compare your answers in soft, sexy, private tones.

---

You may also want to employ some "tools for touch" in your explorations. For example, being caressed by a hand covered with fine, silky material can increase sensual pleasure, as can wearing sheer lingerie. Use of scented oils and creams can be especially sensual as well.

There are various ways to be creative in using tools for touch. For some, the idea of erotically applying whipped cream or chocolate syrup to their partner's body and then luxuriously licking it off might seem too wild. But the bottom line is that what's physically and emotionally safe, what pleases you and your partner, and what you both fully agree on, is what's right for you. The creative and safe use of various materials to enhance touch is something that might at least be fun for you to talk about.

Whether your explorations on an erotic touch date go beyond touch is up to you. As a reminder, to set the most relaxed mood, simply make it your goal to enjoy being together while touching with no necessity to move toward orgasm. For some couples, however, their erotic explorations may lead to one partner genitally manipulating the other, or to mutual masturbation, and they may decide to continue until climax. That's their—and your—decision. However be aware of the possibility that your partner's achieving orgasm may tend to shorten your other exploratory activities.

Much the same can be said about intercourse. Though intercourse will not usually be a specific objective of a date focused on erotic touch, if it turns out that touch exploration naturally leads the couple to desire intercourse, then that's up to them. It's important, however, that this is something *both* partners fully agree on. If one partner wants to keep to the plan of exploring sensual touch, then it is usually preferable for the other to respectfully defer to that partner's wishes.

Whatever you may discover on *your* erotic touch date, it's a good idea for the two of you to talk about it afterward and go over what you've learned about touching each other. What did you discover about what each of you likes? Did you learn anything about painful areas that you didn't know before? Have you found new pleasures in sensual touch that you can take forward into your future sexual relations? This conversation might be a good time for you to set up another erotic touch date.

Probably the best place to have the conversation is in bed at the end of your date. Continuing with the same metaphor from earlier about treating erotic touch as an appetizer, notice that touch—both bonding and erotic—can also serve as a scrumptious dessert as the couple lays in bed talking, intermixing with touching, fondling, stroking, and kissing, perhaps head on shoulder or legs wrapped around each other. Dessert so sweet.

# Chapter Ten

# The Arrow of Romance

Like appreciation, romance between partners often fades over time. Most couples begin with strong romantic feelings when they find themselves in the first blush of love and desire. But once they have been together for a while and the practicalities of life grow more pressing, the romantic element typically weakens. In time, romance may become totally absent from the partnership, even abandoning the playground in the bedroom. If chronic pain enters the picture, the lack of romance may become even more entrenched in the relationship. For the great majority of us, there is nothing more unromantic than pain. Romance is a wellspring of sensual enjoyment, while pain blunts the senses and overrides pleasure. Romance tends to be relaxing and sexually stimulating, while pain is stressful and emotionally harrowing.

Because romance and pain are so opposed, partners facing Cupid's Challenge may feel that being romantic in the bedroom is too much to expect of themselves. However, rekindling romance need not be difficult if partners approach it with an affirmative attitude. And the payoff can be substantial when their efforts heat up their sex life.

How are you and your partner doing in the romance department these days? Does romance still have a solid place in your relationship? Are you using it as a natural way to create more scintillating sex? If your answer is no to either question, then feel comforted knowing that sharpening The Arrow of Romance can help immensely in addressing Cupid's Challenge.

## The Nature of Romance

A good way to begin this part of our journey is to get a clearer understanding of what romance is all about. Of course, different people find different things they consider to be romantic. Still, we can all probably agree on what kinds of activities capture the essence of romance. For instance, consider these scenes:

- Two partners are preparing to go out for a special evening together when the man presents the woman with a single red rose as a token of his love.
- A young man and woman are on a twilight sleigh ride through falling snow, basking in each other's warmth as they sit side by side. They enjoy the hush of the evening, disturbed only by the horse's snow-crunching steps and the sound of sleigh bells. Later, at a wayside inn, they share a cup of hot chocolate by a roaring fire.
- As a husband and wife dance to their favorite song, she lightly caresses his hair while he, captured by her perfume, holds her close and whispers in her ear that he loves her.

There are a few factors in these scenarios that make them so quintessentially romantic. First, in each one, the lovers are sharing an experience marked by emotional togetherness. Second, a main feature of each experience is the pleasurable stimulation of several of the partners' senses. It's the union of the emotional togetherness and the pleasurable stimulation that makes the scenes so romantic. In fact, these two features seem to be central to most romantic experiences.

---

Cupid's Point

Think of an especially romantic experience that you and your partner have had together. What was it that made the experience so romantic? Did you feel especially close to your partner while it was happening?

What were the sensual aspects of the event? Think of each of the five senses—sight, sound, touch, smell, and taste—and write down how each was stimulated during the experience. Was there one sensual aspect that was the most pronounced, or did all of your senses work together to create an overall sensual experience?

---

Good sex, too, is typically about sensory pleasure and emotional closeness. This helps to explain why romantic experiences tend to heighten sexual desire. If you are a woman, you probably understand quite well what I mean. For most women, feeling emotionally close to their partner and enjoying multifaceted sensory pleasures are aspects of the most satisfying sexual experiences. Generally speaking, for women sex and romance naturally go together.

It's different for many, though certainly not for all men. If you are a man reading this, you may be nodding your head in agreement when I say that rekindling romance is a great way to improve your and your partner's sex life. However, if you're still not sold on the idea of romance, just give it a chance. If you do, I think you'll find it to be one of your most effective approaches for managing the effects of chronic pain on your sex life.

With that said, let's find out what steps you and your partner can take to kindle romance.

## Creating a Romantic Atmosphere in Your Bedroom

It stands to reason that an excellent way to increase the level of romance in your bedroom is to create an atmosphere that heightens sensual pleasure. Ideally, lovers stimulate and please all five of their senses. We've already talked at length about touch. So that leaves four others: sight, sound, smell, and taste.

There are some specific ways you can stimulate each of these senses in the bedroom. But the overall idea is to create a bedroom that is a comfortable, romantic haven for you and your partner. For many who must deal with persistent pain, the bedroom unfortunately tends to gradually evolve into a kind of sickroom, with bottles of pills and various ointments piled on the side table and with an overall atmosphere, including perhaps even with smells, of a place thats main purpose is for convalescence. It's easy to imagine how an environment like this can make it difficult to get into a sexy mood, so it's important to try to ensure that your bedroom doesn't become just a place where you or your partner go when you aren't feeling well. Instead, make it an inviting hideaway where the two of you can "get it on" in comfortable, sexy surroundings that appeal to your sensual natures.

## Sight

One of the most effective ways to create a more pleasing sensory atmosphere in your bedroom is to pay close attention to what you see. When you walk into the room, do you see clutter that makes you want to turn around and walk back out? Does the bed beckon to you, seeming to beg you and your partner to climb in? How about the light in the bedroom, and the colors? Are those pleasing to your eyes? In order to create a bedroom that tempts the senses, it's not necessary to strive for something out of *Architectural Digest*. Nor is a large space necessary. A small, simple, well-kept bedroom can be visually pleasing, and can virtually whisper intimacy and sensuality.

Put in the right kind of light. Vision begins with light. In many relationships, one or both partners prefer to have sex with the light on so they can see and visually enjoy each other. But if the light is too glaring, it can detract from the lovers' visual pleasure. The problem is easily remedied by making sure that there are one or two lamps in the bedroom with lights that can be adjusted to create a softer or brighter ambience to satisfy your and your lover's desires.

A few candles can also help create a romantic mood by the flickering light and shadows they create. If the candles are scented, they may do double sensual duty. But if you use scented candles, make sure both of you like the fragrance and strength.

Cleanliness and neatness are basic. A messy bedroom, with clutter on the bed, dresser, chair, or floor—or even worse, a bedroom that obviously needs a good scrubbing—can grate on the eyes. To make your bedroom special, begin with keeping it clean and neat. Get out the vacuum and the dust cloth if needed, and tidy up any clutter. Pick up the kids' toys that have somehow found their way through your bedroom door and return them to their proper place. And make sure the bed is made, even if you and your partner are soon going to be unmaking it. Don't wait for a sexy feeling to wash over the two of you before taking care of these basics. That way when a sultry mood strikes, you won't have to put it on hold to first straighten up the bedroom.

Let your eye be your guide. Peruse your bedroom from various perspectives. Do the colors and textures please your senses? Could it be time for a little redecorating? Often, very little effort and expense are required to create a more visually pleasing atmosphere, one with shape, color, texture, and light that beckon partners to enjoy one another. Making a few small changes such as putting a couple of extra pillows on the bed or purchasing new curtains can help create a romantic mood for you and your mate.

What you wear can make a difference. At home, many of us feel most comfortable in old sweats, a favorite flannel nightgown, or a T-shirt and threadbare jeans. Be aware, however, that the clothes you tend to relax in may not put your lover into a sexy frame of mind. For women, donning a negligee or some other sheer, revealing piece of clothing before bed may go a long way toward pleasing her partner and making her feel more sexy herself. Much the same goes for men. Many a male has found that the simple act of putting on a pair of silky boxers before bed can stimulate the sexual interest of both his mate and himself.

---

Cupid's Point

What other changes in the visual aspects of your bedroom might help create a more romantic atmosphere? For example, might a well-placed painting or two on the walls make the space more pleasant? Or is there a television set in your bedroom that is too often turned on when you and your partner might instead be enjoying each other's company more intimately?

Think about each of the other senses discussed in the text and how your bedroom atmosphere might be changed to allow for fuller stimulation of those senses. For instance, how could you better cultivate the sense of touch in your bedroom?

Ask your partner these same questions to find out how he or she thinks your bedroom atmosphere might be altered to become more sensation-friendly.

---

It's a good idea to talk with your partner about what you would like to see each other wear to bed. If the idea of wearing what your partner likes makes you uncomfortable, it's all right to say that. At the same time, remember that stretching yourself a bit can sometimes lead to exciting progress. Maybe those silky boxers will feel good once you try them on. Or perhaps that little bit of satin that leaves hardly anything to the imagination will make you feel so sexy that you can barely keep your hands off yourself, let alone your partner!

## Sound

Blocking out the outside world. It can be difficult to make your bedroom into a sensual haven if noise from the street or from family members in other parts of the house is constantly impinging. But for most of us, tearing down the walls and rebuilding our bedroom with extra sound-proofing is out of the question. There are, however, some relatively simple steps that you can take to help insulate your bedroom from unwanted noise. One method, if you have an audio system or even a smartphone app available in your bedroom, is to play ocean, tropical, or other natural sounds that can help block out the external distractions while helping to create a relaxed, romantic mood.

Another way to counteract unwanted sound is to use a fan or an air purifier to create white noise. This may be an effective alternative unless the device has to be turned up so loud that it becomes disturbing in itself. Also, be careful that the soft, calming sound doesn't lull you to sleep before the festivities begin!

Perhaps the most effective way for you and your partner to lessen the impact of external noise is to lose yourselves in your sighs and vocalizations of pleasure. Once you get to that point, other noises tend to fade into the background.

Music. Romantic sounds playing in the background over your audio system can be a powerful mood enhancer too. This is definitely an area where the input of both partners is needed because music that one thinks is romantic and sexy may be quite different from what the other likes. By talking it over, the two of you can probably find areas of agreement about what sets a sensual mood.

Soft music can also be used to signal your partner that you are in the mood for romance. It's a way of gently encouraging and instigating a romantic encounter.

Talk. A few well-placed words between partners can often be intensely romantic and sensual. Remember the earlier scene in which the husband whispers "I love you" to his wife while they are dancing? Well, his words would be even more romantic and powerful if he were to utter them while they were enjoying sex together.

Many couples say little to each other in bed because they've never done so and don't know where to start. But telling each other how you feel is not all that hard. It's often just a matter of making a small appreciative comment while you are touching, kissing, or doing whatever you are doing. For instance:

- "You feel so good to me."
- "You look hot in that negligee."
- "You're still the only man for me."
- "I'm hard as a rock for you."
- "You make me feel like a twenty-year-old."

What a delectable, sense-heightening joy such words can bring for the recipient. Plus the feedback the giver receives is often immediate and unmistakably positive. It's fairly easy to start with a few simple words such as those above, and go from there knowing there's plenty of room for growth.

## Smell

Cleanliness and natural smells. The sensual power unleashed by the sense of smell begins with cleanliness. Fortunately, most of us realize that cleanliness adds to both our partner's and our own sexual experience, not least because it's a way of showing mutual respect. This isn't to say that sandblasting your body is necessary before engaging in sex. Many men and women appreciate the natural smell of their partner. But a quick shower or bath just before going to bed, or the efficient use of a wet wash cloth or towel, is a way for partners to show love and respect for each other as well as to freshen themselves. For some, a long, leisurely bath before bed can be an especially powerful way to arouse sensuality. Of course, taking that bath or shower together may be even more arousing!

Perfumes and other added scents. Our sense of smell is intimately related to a primitive part of our brain linking to our emotions. That may be why a certain scent can powerfully evoke a particular time in our life and how we felt back then. It may also help explain why perfumes, colognes, and various lotions and creams can have a strong effect on the libido. Wearing a well-chosen perfume or cologne may be one of your most powerful ways to romanticize the mood and arouse your partner's senses."Well-chosen" means a scent that your partner likes. Ladies, it may take a little persistence and gentle prodding of your partner to get feedback on what he prefers. Be patient though and try to find that special perfume that turns his head right to you.

For men, you too can play this enjoyable game of finding a scent that pleases your mate. You can often depend on the salesperson behind a store's aromatics counter for some advice on cologne or aftershave. But your best guide is your partner and her responsiveness to you.

## Taste_

Romantic dinners. The popularity of movies such as *Eat Drink Man Woman* and *Chocolat* testify to the close connection between food and sensuality. Stimulating the sense of taste to enhance a romantic atmosphere is not about gorging ourselves so that we fall asleep the moment we hit the bed. But rather it's about preparing and eating nutritionally sound meals that fulfill our health requirements, awaken our taste buds, and provide us with energy—all of which help to put us into a sexy mood.

It's also about the setting in which we enjoy the meal. Whether you go out to a nice restaurant or prepare a special dinner at home for just the two of you, the food and the setting should work together to create the kind of romantic mood that leads you and your partner naturally to the bedroom. That means your other senses should also be brought into play. Your eyes can be engaged by the ambience of the restaurant and the way the meal is visually presented. If you stay home (hopefully, with any children able to stay with their grandparents for the night), your visual sense can be heightened by the way you prepare your dining room. For example, you might turn down the overhead lights and switch on a soft lamp or light a few candles.

Being together for a special occasion can also be sexually heightened through visuals, for instance by you and your partner dressing nicely even if you remain at home. This doesn't mean a formal gown, a tux, or even a suit. But for him, shaving and putting on a clean shirt, and for her, donning one of her favorite outfits, can add to the feeling that the dinner is something out of the ordinary. The couple can create an exciting variation if she wears some sheer piece of intimate apparel and he a short robe with a pair of nice boxers—or perhaps nothing—beneath. Remember, however, to move the food and utensils away before using the table for anything other than eating. (And make sure the table is very sturdy!)

Romantic music playing in the background during your meal can add to the sensual mood as well. What you talk about is also important. Leave the problems at work for another conversation and realize that a romantic get-together can provide a natural setting for an appreciation date in which you focus on celebrating your partnership and each other.

Whatever the specifics, make the dinner a memorable occasion in which several of your senses are brought into play. It's difficult to go right away from a nice dinner back into the routine of everyday life, so hopefully you won't immediately return to the living room just to turn the television on. Instead, gravitate into the bedroom and complete the evening in intimate style.

## Building Romance through Sharing Special Experiences

Creating an atmosphere that pleasurably stimulates you and your partner's senses is only one aspect of building a more romantic relationship. As we learned earlier, romance is also about feeling emotionally close to one another. As a result, another way to make romance a larger part of your relationship is to increase your connection to your partner. And not just in the bedroom.

Feeling emotionally close isn't something a couple can turn on and off depending on whether or not they're engaged in sexual activities. If partners often feel distant from one another, that state of mind is unlikely to go away just because it's time for bed. Closeness is something that occurs within the wholeness of the relationship.

What Creates Emotional Intimacy

Partners grow emotionally close to one another for many reasons. Working together to build a home, creating a family, facing problems as a couple, helping each other—all of these and many other factors may contribute to a couple's sense that they have an intimate bond.

One of the most important contributors to feeling closely connected is the sharing of special experiences. For most couples such experiences begin with dating; when being together becomes an overriding goal in the budding relationship. These special experiences may eventually culminate in one of the most memorable events in the partners' lives—the wedding ceremony—which is often followed by another exceptional event, the honeymoon.

Unfortunately, as the relationship moves on, and this also pertains to couples who stay together even if they don't get married, the early flood of shared special experiences often diminishes to a trickle. If that happens, then even if the partners are striving for similar goals, they may feel increasingly emotionally distant from one another. That distance is partly caused by a lack of new bonding experiences like those that had previously drawn them close when their relationship was young, such as the sense that they were on an adventure together sharing the sweetness of life and making memories as a couple. But in the present they share so few special experiences that they feel they are walking down different roads, or living in different worlds.

This is a common story, and a sad one. However, it provides a good lesson by clarifying a principle that couples can use to draw closer and rekindle romance. The principle is this: to become emotionally closer, share more special experiences together.

"Special" experiences do not need to be totally out of the ordinary. And you and your partner don't have to take out a second mortgage so you can go on a trip around the world!

Of course, special experiences *may* include rare or once in a lifetime happenings. But more importantly, they may be everyday events such as going to a movie, taking a walk together, or keeping a morning ritual of sharing a cup of coffee. These "everyday" special events can serve just as well as the more exceptional ones. That's because what truly makes a shared experience special is the attitude the partners take toward it. The main thing that's required is simply that they enjoy each other's company as they experience some aspect of life together.

---

Cupid's Point

Make a list of the everyday special activities that you and your partner engage in such as going to movies or concerts, for drives in the country, or for walks. Do those activities refresh your partnership and build closeness? Do they make a difference in your enjoyment of sex? Are there any everyday special activities that you seldom or never do that you would like to experience with your partner?

If you are living with chronic pain, does it limit the everyday special activities you can do? Does your condition truly limit you, or is the limitation more in the form of a mindset? If the former, consider asking your physician for advice about everyday special activities that you and your partner could enjoy together. If the latter, how might you change the mindset?

---

All couples need everyday special times together. Such experiences are one of the main nurturers of a relationship. Sharing special times is especially important for couples who are beset by chronic pain. It not only draws partners closer together, it tends to pick up the spirits of the one dealing with chronic pain while keeping him or her active in the world. In that way, it counteracts the tendency of those who live with recurring pain to hide themselves in their house or apartment, not wanting to engage with the outside world any more than necessary. The other member of the couple may even fall into the same pattern. But when partners keep the door to the outside world closed, they miss out on countless opportunities to experience the joy of life singularly as well as together.

If the one living with pain is severely limited in locomotive ability, a little extra thought may be needed to determine appropriate special activities to share. If he or she is bedridden, for example, then it's time to be inventive. Almost always, there will still be entertaining ways for the couple to share special times. For instance, by playing card games or watching movies together. With lots of talk and laughter, and with love and good feelings permeating the relationship, such occasions can be memorable and help the couple bond more tightly together.

The key point here is that almost any shared activity that serves to break up the sameness of day-to-day living can be a special experience; an opportunity for the two of you to enjoy life together.

But isn't it unrealistic, some might ask, to expect partners who are facing the daily problems and deadlines of making a living, taking care of the house, and caring for kids or other family members to find the time for special get-togethers? And isn't it even worse for those who are facing Cupid's Challenge? After all, dealing with chronic pain itself can be a dominant issue.

No, it's not unrealistic. What's unrealistic is to expect that a partnership, whether beset by chronic pain or not, will thrive without such experiences. It's a matter of choice. The choice has to do with the quality of life that partners want. These shared experiences are ones that make life sweet, joyful, and worth living. So a critical decision for all couples is whether they are going to strive for a relationship in which they make time to enjoy the world together and grow closer to each other—and that includes couples who are facing Cupid's Challenge. There is no reason for partners who are facing the problem of persistent pain to accept a lower quality of life than other couples, though naturally a healthy respect for limitations needs to be taken into account.

By finding ways to create special experiences and build romance in your partnership, you will be choosing to meet Cupid's Challenge head-on by sweetening your life in and out of the bedroom.

## Romance, Attitude, Light, and Appreciation

Though romance belongs in the sensual dimension of Cupid's Challenge because it involves sensual experience, it's also true that romance involves partners' attitudes toward each other which involves the psychological dimension. But if romance is also a matter of attitude, that means the Arrow of Romance is closely related to the Arrow of Attitude.

So when partners increase the level of romance in their relationship, they also tend to create a more affirmative attitude toward each other, their sexuality, their partnership, and their power to deal with chronic pain. It's not difficult to understand why this happens when we realize that the presence of romance within a relationship constitutes an affirmation of the couple's love. For example, when a man brings his partner flowers, he is affirming her value to him. Similarly, when a woman kisses her mate sweetly, she is affirming his value to her. In both cases, they are at the same time affirming their relationship. The same goes for when partners increase romance by making sure they have "ordinary" special times to spend together.

The Arrow of Romance is also closely related to the Arrow of Light. Earlier we focused on how for most of us sex was at first a wonderful, exciting ecstasy. But over time we may have lost some of the sense of playfulness and pleasurableness, especially when living with chronic pain. Notice how romance, however, is itself a kind of lightness. So it stands to reason that one of the best ways for couples to prevent a sense of heaviness from permeating their bedroom or other parts of their relationship as they deal with Cupid's Challenge is to increase their romance quotient.

Finally, the Arrow of Romance is also a friend to the Arrow of Appreciation. After all, romantic words and actions are often expressions of appreciation. For instance, when a man presents his partner with flowers, he is demonstrating his appreciation of her. When a woman kisses her mate, she is showing her affection for him, which is a way of acknowledging her appreciation of him. Special occasions is also a way for partners to appreciate each other. For a couple to go for a walk together in the evening after dinner is not only romantic, it's a way for them to show their regard for one another.

Put it all together and it's as plain and as sweet as the fragrance of a rose: romance is one of Cupid's most precious and useful tools.

# Chapter Eleven

# The Arrow of Innovation

Progress requires change. In fact, progress *is* change. It stands to reason that achieving a happier sex life while managing chronic pain may require you and your partner to make some changes in areas of your lives such as lifestyle, attitude, and communication. Another area in which adaptation is likely to be necessary is in your bedroom activities. To address Cupid's Challenge most effectively, you may need to do old things in new ways in bed, or even try new things that you have never done before.

For some, making that kind of change can be a little scary because it takes them out of their comfort zone. They may balk at the idea of trying something unfamiliar, preferring to stay with what's "tried and true." But that's just the point. If the customary ways of behaving in the bedroom are no longer working, then they are no longer tried and true.

That's where the Arrow of Innovation comes in. Innovation is about you and your partner exploring new ways of relating to each other sexually. It's a wonderful approach because new practices and techniques often serve two functions: not only can they reduce pain levels, they can also help the two of you to increase your eroticism and discover pleasures you have never experienced before.

The methods and activities are not particularly esoteric or unusual. Most couples will already be aware of some or all of them. But that's not to say they practice them. For many couples, sex is synonymous with intercourse, and for them intercourse happens in only one way.

## Making Intercourse Enjoyable Again

For many relationships, the most troublesome aspect of Cupid's Challenge is how to have pain-free intercourse. Painful intercourse is often associated with joint or skeletal problems such as arthritis or low back pain. But there are also numerous other culprits, including skin oversensitivity and recurrent pelvic pain.

For some individuals intercourse is not advisable until the condition has been adequately treated or even totally alleviated. This is something that should be determined by your physician (or, if it's your partner's pain, by his or her physician). With your doctor's go-ahead, there are often definitive steps that you and your loved one can take to lessen any discomfort associated with intercourse.

### Position Yourselves for Success

Pain can often be greatly alleviated if partners simply change the position in which they have intercourse. This is especially true for pain that originates from joint or skeletal conditions. The missionary position, with the man on top of the woman, partly supporting his weight by his arms and shoulders, is still the main approach for having intercourse. Perhaps this was the way the lovers first enjoyed sex together and it became habitual. However, it may not be the optimal arrangement for couples facing Cupid's Challenge due to the strain it can place on both participants.

That strain can be considerable. For one thing, the partial weight of her partner pressing down can cause undue stress on the woman's muscles, joints, and other skeletal elements. She is also somewhat restricted in her movements in the missionary position, which can contribute to additional discomfort, especially if her flexibility has been compromised by her condition.

The man, too, may find the missionary position troublesome by his having to support himself. Not just his arms and shoulders, but his wrists, back, hips, and legs are typically involved in preventing his weight from bearing down too heavily on his partner. If he has joint or lower back problems, the position can cause unwanted stress that aggravates those conditions and leads to fatigue and pain.

To continue using the missionary position even when it results in pain doesn't make a lot of sense—not even if "that's the way we've always done it." There are other positions that are generally less stressful on joints and muscles, and these may provide every bit as much sensory stimulation. In some cases, even more. Four such arrangements follow.

Lying sideways, face-to-face. This is the missionary position moved ninety degrees in one direction or the other so that the partners are lying on their sides, facing each other. This position has several advantages over the man-on-top position by serving to reduce stress that might cause undue discomfort. First, the position allows the partners to arrange themselves so that there is little or no excess weight on the woman to press against her muscles, joints, and frame. Also, she generally has greater freedom of movement in this position, being better able to arrange her limbs and torso comfortably. For the man, lying on his side does not require him to use his arms and back to support himself as he fights against the pull of gravity. This usually results in considerably less stress on his body. Like his partner, the man tends to have greater freedom of movement while lying on his side too, and it's easier for him to find a comfortable arrangement of his limbs and torso in which to gain maximum erotic contact with his lover. All of this makes the position especially appropriate for an assortment of conditions that can cause chronic pain.

Spooning. In this position, so named because it's analogous to two spoons, one nestled within the other, the lovers lie on their sides with the man's chest facing the woman's back, as he enters her from behind. The spooning position has many of the same advantages of the sideways, face-to-face position, in that it reduces weight and stress on both partners' bodies and allows for greater freedom of movement. Use of a pillow between the woman's knees may further help reduce stress on her hips, knees, and legs.

The spooning position has several advantages from the stand-point of sensuality. For one thing, it takes little effort for the man's hands to reach and stimulate his partner's breasts and nipples in this arrangement, something that may be very pleasurable to both. Also, given the placement of the man's arms and hands, it is usually a rela-tively simple matter for him to reach down and stimulate his partner's clitoris from the front. For many women, such stimulation can add greatly to pleasure during intercourse.

Some may think that a degree of intimacy is lost in the spooning position because the partners are not facing each other. However, it has the advantage that the man is typically in a perfect place to speak softly to his partner about his love and desire. As we learned, a few well-placed words during sex can greatly add to sensuality in the bed-room, and spooning makes it easy for the man to do so.

Woman lying on her back, man standing. If the couple's bed is high enough in relation to the man's height, this may be, especially for the woman, a relatively stress-free position that helps increase variety in the bedroom. The woman lies on her back with her buttocks near the edge of the bed, while her partner stands between her legs holding them up in a comfortable position. Alternatively, the woman may place her legs on her partner's shoulders or around his waist. The advantage of such an arrangement for the female partner is the absence of pressure from above and having her legs well supported, especially if they are held by her partner or rest on his shoulders.

For many men this may be a relatively comfortable position too because it allows a good deal of freedom of movement. The man can gain support for his legs by bracing them against the bed. However, the position does require adequate leg and hip strength for the male partner and may put unacceptably high stress on his knees if the bed is not sufficiently high.

Man lying on his back, woman sitting on top, facing. For many partners, this is an enjoyable and comfortable position, especially when reducing stress on the male partner's frame is important. Downward pressure on the man may be minimized by the woman leaning forward to partly support her weight on her arms and legs. However, the position may not be as comfortable for the woman for that very reason, or if bent knees tend to cause undue physical stress. Use of strategically placed pillows under the man's back, hips, or legs may further enhance his comfort. Notably, many women, and often men too, relish the idea of the female being on top; something that they might not be accustomed to. In particular, she may like being in greater control of the movements during intercourse than she would be in some other positions, and the man may enjoy lying back while his partner determines the rhythm of movements.

A variation on this position is for the man to sit in an armless chair with the woman on his lap facing him. She places her arms around his neck or shoulders, her legs splayed out on each side, her feet meeting the floor to provide support for moving up and down. A very sturdy chair is mandatory, one that can easily hold the weight of both partners as they move, and it is essential that both partners' balance be maintained at all times. For some couples, a large armchair can work well. However, since this may require the woman's knees to be up and bent, it may not be appropriate for some.

---

Cupid's Point

If you and your partner engage in intercourse, do you simply follow past practice, or do you go with the flow of the moment? Is it something you explicitly talk about?

Do any of the illustrated positions seem like they might be especially appropriate for you and your partner, or perhaps inappropriate given your situation? Can you think of any other positions that have worked or might work well for you in reducing pain and providing pleasure?

Experimenting with positions for intercourse to reduce pain and increase sensuality can afford an excellent opportunity for you and your partner to apply *ICE*:

- First, identify just what is causing discomfort during inter-course. Who is uncomfortable and how much? What is it about your current position that leads to the problem?
- Second, talk about alternative positions and what each of you finds most appealing about them. Do any of them look like they might substantially alleviate the problem? Which ones may also heighten the sensual aspects of intercourse? Choose one or more positions that seem most likely to help reduce discomfort.
- Third, actually explore the positions you chose. How do they work in practice for you? Which does each partner find most comfortable? Which brings the most sensual delight to both of you?

Understand that even positions as relatively stress-free as lying sideways face-to-face, and spooning can have drawbacks in some cases. For example, lying on their side even on a comfortable bed may aggravate hip problems for some. The basic rules are to use good sense, communicate clearly, seek both partners' comfort, and stay safe. Be sure to enlist your doctor's advice on the matter. He or she should know your condition intimately and be able to advise you on which positions will give you your best opportunity to minimize pain and discomfort.

### Dealing with Vaginal Dryness

If the female partner's natural bodily lubrication is low so that pain results when the male inserts his penis, be gentle in your understand-ing of what this is due to. One of the most common reasons is sim-ply that she is lacking in sexual desire at the time when insertion is attempted. If that's the reason, it's important for the partners to dis-cuss how they can better relate sexually. In some cases the basic problem is that the man moves too fast into intercourse, not allowing his partner sufficient time to warm up to being more receptive. This can often be resolved fairly easily through clear, caring communication and the will to work together to seek solutions.

For many women, even sexual excitement does not lead to adequate lubrication. In some of these cases hormone therapy can have beneficial results. In others, the use of personal, water-based lubricants may help eliminate unwanted friction and enable enjoyable intercourse.

One patient confided in me that she and her husband had made the application of this kind of lubricant a main feature in their sexual trysts. Her husband used his fingers to liberally apply the lubricant—a water-based cream made specifically for that purpose—to her vagina and surrounding areas as she lay back and luxuriated in his touch. She said that her husband enjoyed intimately touching her and discovering her reactions. She then experienced what she called "heavenly" sensations that usually resulted in at least one orgasm. The extended foreplay, she told me, consistently led to pain-free and very satisfying intercourse for both.

So, guys take note! And women too, because my patient also told me that a variation on the theme was for her to apply the same lubricant to her husband. She said that the results of doing so had sometimes proved to be, in her word, "sizzling!"

## Other Intercourse Inhibitors
Painful intercourse can arise from a number of other conditions. Two of the more common complaints are vulvar pain and pain caused by a tightening of the vaginal muscles (vaginismus). There can be several sources of the former, but occasionally it is the result of something as simple as irritation caused by washing the area with plain soap. As for the latter, tightening of the vaginal muscles may have both physical and psychological precursors. Your primary physician or gynecologist can best advise you.

Overall, whenever pain arises in intercourse, whether it's chronic or only occasional, whether you're a man or a woman, if you are feeling pain of any sort during intercourse talk to your physician about it as soon as possible. Your doctor can then advise you about proper treatment and whether continued intercourse and under what conditions is advisable. If your physician says go ahead, then don't let old habits block you from exploring new lovemaking positions that add comfort and sensuality.

## Variety, the Spice of Love

Scintillating sex can be so much more than intercourse as you learn to cultivate all five senses in your lovemaking. In addition, there are a number of other specific activities that can provide erotic diversity. Some of these can be especially appropriate for partners facing Cupid's Challenge because they are relatively pain-free and have considerable power to heat up the bedroom. This makes them just the kind of activity that Cupid favors.

Not everyone will see them that way though. Some may feel that these sexual activities are not for them. And maybe they're right. But be careful not to pass judgment too quickly. Sexuality and intimacy can take many pleasurable forms and we shortchange ourselves if we decide we won't like something, especially before even trying it. So give variety a chance in your bedroom! Spice is important to erotic love as well as to life in general.

<u>Oral Sex</u>

Going on the basis of articles in some women's magazines geared to the would-be sophisticate, you might come to the conclusion that every adult in our society is a frequent practitioner of oral sex. By "oral sex" I mean a man's oral contact with his lover's vaginal area or a woman's oral contact with her lover's penis and/or testicles. But this proclaimed popularity is not all together true as there remain many individuals who have either never engaged in such activities, or have tried oral sex a few times and decided it was not for them. As a result, many relationships, including those facing Cupid's Challenge, are devoid of oral sex.

This is unfortunate for a couple of reasons. First, performing oral sex is usually physically undemanding of partners. Second, many couples find this kind of activity to be one of the most pleasurable parts of their sex lives.

Performing fellatio is physically undemanding because the contact that occurs between one partner's mouth and the other's genitals can take place in a great number of positions. This usually makes it comparatively easy for partners to find a comfortable arrangement of their bodies for engaging in oral sex. When the recipient is female, inserting a pillow under her buttocks so as to raise her pelvic area may enhance the comfort and pleasure of both partners. Of course, when lovers engage in mutual oral sex simultaneously, in the so-called 69 position, they may have fewer positioning options.

One reason many couples find oral sex to be so enjoyable is that it involves one or both of the lovers focusing very specifically on what is usually the most erogenous zone of their partner's body. When mouth, lips, and tongue—with all their warmth and moisture—are applied to these erogenous zones, powerfully erotic sensations may result for the lovers.

A second factor making oral sex pleasurable is that lips, tongue, and even teeth (used very gently) can often be applied with great precision to please your mate sensually. In performing cunnilingus, her lover may fine-tune his efforts to stimulate her clitoris in the exact way that gives her optimum pleasure. This may also involve the use of his hands and fingers. For example, he may use his thumb and forefinger to separate his partner's labia majora (outer lips) for direct access with his lips and tongue to her typically very sensitive clitoris. The female partner, too, may be able to provide very specific sensual pleasure to her mate through the precise use of her mouth, tongue, teeth, and hands.

We shouldn't be surprised that fellatio can be so stimulating. The oral cavity, along with its parts, is exceedingly versatile. This is shown by the fact that the vast range of sounds made in spoken human languages is largely the result of different positionings of the lips, tongue, teeth, and palate. If the mouth can produce so many distinct languages, then it can certainly be used with great versatility too in producing the language of sensual love when partners orally please each other.

Not only the recipient, but also the giver can derive great pleasure from oral sex. When the giver becomes aware that he or she is providing intense pleasure to his or her partner, this knowledge may be highly erotic in itself. A kind of synergistic effect may then occur, with the giver redoubling his efforts and his mate being the beneficiary of even greater enjoyment. Because of its powerful effect, many couples also find oral sex to be an excellent aid to intercourse by helping to restore the male partner's hardness in the event that he loses his erection.

Another reason oral sex can be pleasing to both recipient and giver is that it is such an intimate activity. Some couples feel that oral sex is the most intimate thing that they do together and that it unites them sensually and sexually more completely than any other sex act. This helps make it a most effective part of the Arrow of Innovation. When the object is to maximize erotic love, oral sex is one of Cupid's favorite approaches.

Still, oral sex strikes some people as "dirty." They may look at the genital area of their partner, and of themselves, as being somehow fundamentally unclean. Whether this belief stems from childhood admonitions or some other source, it can lead the individual to consider oral sex to be unhygienic. But it is not innately so. The genital area is simply another part of our bodies and is not by its nature "unclean." For the great majority of couples, if partners thoroughly wash and dry those parts of their bodies prior to sexual activity, oral sex is as sanitary, and in some cases more so, than kissing on the mouth. To help add to their mutual aesthetic and sensual pleasure during oral sex, some couples make it a practice to keep their pubic areas trimmed, or for the woman, waxed completely. Of course, partners may also trim or shave one another's pubic areas adding yet another sensual element to their activities.

It is important to clarify that when a woman performs oral sex on her lover she does not need to receive his semen in her mouth. When this is an issue, it is best that the partners discuss it with an open mind. If the woman decides she does not want to do so, her mate needs to honor her wishes without blame and make sure he withdraws before ejaculating.

You and your partner may have already discovered the pleasures of oral sex. If not, and if you feel it's time to consider adding it to your sexual activities, then a good way to begin, as always, is with communication. If either partner has qualms, discuss them. You may need some time. Neither partner should feel rushed or pressured into engaging in this, or in any other kind of sexual activity. Of course, caring communication should always be your objective in such discussions.

A natural place to talk about the subject is in bed. That way, if the two of you decide to move forward in your exploration, you can do so at that moment if the mood is right. You may want to start slowly with an intimate kiss or a flick of the tongue to get your bearings. Understand that ideally, oral sex will be a mutual activity with both partners acting as giver and receiver at different times, or at the same time. However, this is not set in stone. It may work best for you and your lover for only one to be the giver and one the recipient. That's for you to talk about and decide.

Be sure to stay patient with one another and to keep communicating. If you are the giver, seek feedback from your partner about what you are doing. If you are the recipient and your partner does something to make you feel especially good, let him or her know realizing that your sighs and bodily movements may be ambiguous. The clearest communication is to explicitly say what feels good, such as:

"Mmmm. That was nice. Please do that again."

"Can you do it just like that, except up just a little?...Yes, right there."

---

Cupid's Point

Clear feedback is essential if partners are to understand what most pleases each other. Yet, as we have discussed earlier, many partners find it difficult to articulate how they feel in bed.

How well do you and your partner provide each other with feedback while you are engaged in sexual activities? Is your feedback mostly nonverbal, for example with sighs and movements? Or do you articulate how you feel in clear language? Can you think of things you might say in bed to add to the sexy atmosphere?

---

## Mutual Masturbation

Another important aspect of sensual touch is masturbation, especially mutual masturbation.

Most of us learn about masturbation fairly early in life, and for many—both men and women—it is a practice that continues into adulthood. Masturbation in the form of manipulating one's own genitals for the purpose of gratification is often an important means of sexual relief, especially for individuals who are not in a relationship. But self-masturbation can also provide much more than relief. It can be quite erotic in itself through discovering more about our sensuality, including where and how we prefer to be sexually touched.

Mutual masturbation can be even more erotic. For partners facing Cupid's Challenge, it offers, like oral sex, the crucial advantage of having fewer physical demands than intercourse. This can make it an appropriate substitute when intercourse is too painful. It may also be used as a supplement to intercourse to provide added sensual variety.

Mutual masturbation has two basic forms. In the first, lovers touch and manipulate their own genital areas, but in the presence of one another. This can be done while lying down, sitting, standing, or in just about any position that the partners find comfortable. It is thus a sexual practice that generally places few demands on frames, joints, and muscles. This is not to say that in all cases it is totally pain-free. For example, there may be some difficulty for those with arthritis or other joint problems that affect the hands or wrists.

Mutual masturbation can take the form of lovers laying side by side, for example, watching one another. They may talk during the activity, asking one another how they feel and describing their own feelings and sensations. Some individuals may feel hesitant at first to allow their partner to see them masturbate. This may be due to them feeling a sense of guilt associated with the act. But when partners do it together, their mutuality tends to alleviate such feelings.

To help further allay potential embarrassment, it may be helpful for the woman to realize that many men consider the idea of female masturbation to be very erotic. They feel that it emphasizes the woman's femininity. Similarly, many women enjoy watching their mate sensually pleasure himself at the same time that she is doing so.

The second kind of mutual masturbation occurs when the lovers manipulate one another's genitals, either consecutively or at the same time. When lovers masturbate one another consecutively, this allows for almost as much freedom in positioning as the first kind of masturbation. But when erotic manipulations occur simultaneously, there is more restriction. Still, even in this case, it is usually relatively easy for partners to find a position that is comfortable for both. They might, for example, lie on their sides face-to- face, or sit together on the bed, their heads and backs amply supported by pillows. One of the most comfortable positions may be to lay feet to head. Note that this position might naturally evolve into or include oral sex.

The kind of sensual touch date we discussed earlier can provide an excellent atmosphere and opportunity for exploring mutual masturbation. In any event, it's wise for partners to create a relaxed, sensual atmosphere as they experiment with mutual masturbation, to be patient with each other, and to remember that their main objective is to enjoy each other's company.

Sexual Aids

Of the various kinds of so-called sex toys—what I call *sensual assistants*—the most predominant are probably penis substitutes. These include vibrators, dildos, and artificial penis extenders. Vibrators and dildos may be especially useful for many couples coping with Cupid's Challenge, especially when the pain problem revolves around joint or other structural issues, as well as for much the same reason that oral sex and mutual masturbation can be valuable—using them is usually less physically demanding than intercourse.

Vibrators and dildos are generally used to stimulate the female partner's clitoris or for vaginal insertion to simulate intercourse. They may be employed by the woman alone or in concert with her mate. Used in the second way, the woman may apply the vibrator or dildo herself while her mate watches her or holds her. Or he may add his own stimulation in several ways, including orally, with his fingers, or with his penis touching her. Alternatively, he may use the instrument to stimulate her.

This form of erotic engagement usually puts relatively little stress on either partner's body and allows both to assume a variety of positions. Such aids though won't serve well if vaginal insertion results in pain, oversensitivity, or irritation. To help reduce that possibility, it is important that there be adequate lubrication whenever a vibrator or dildo is used.

Some may view dildos and vibrators to be somehow unnatural or lewd. A more constructive view is to recognize them as sensual tools that may help reduce discomfort while providing pleasure and enhancing intimacy. Keeping the aids clean is very important. After each use they should be washed well with hot water, thoroughly rinsed, dried, and stored for their next use. Of course, dildos and vibrators can be enjoyed in conjunction with other sexual activities. Some couples find that using them while engaging in oral sex or mutual masturbation, or even intercourse, adds to their overall sexual pleasure.

## Other Tools for Cupid

Another device that some couples use to help enliven their sex life is the camera. Many a woman and man has luxuriated in the "naughtiness" of modeling while their partner plays the role of erotic photographer with a digital or instant camera. The session itself and viewing the finished photographs together may serve as an aphrodisiac for lovers. Of course partners need to take special care to safeguard these photos from any prying eyes.

Though none of these sexy tools reduce pain specifically, they can play an important part in helping lovers offset chronic pain by increasing sensual pleasure. By giving your imagination free reign, perhaps you and your partner can think of other sexual aids that would fit a broader definition to possibly include lighting, candles, music, lingerie, and more as discussed earlier.

Did I hear someone say something about whipped cream? Well, I hope it's the low-fat variety!

---

### Cupid's Point

Can you think of any other physical sexual aids that might help heat up your bedroom? One way to approach this is in terms of the five senses. What visual aids might there be other than wearing sexy clothes to bed? Can you think of any auditory aids other than music and talking to one another? How about other aids for touch? Smell? Taste?

This could be an enjoyable exercise to talk over with your partner. Especially in bed. Let your imaginations roam freely!

---

## Your Most Powerful Sexual Aid

Your most powerful sexual aid in the bedroom is your mind. And that's as true for partners who are dealing with chronic pain as for others. Sadly, too many couples try to be innovative in the bedroom while retaining old, outmoded mindsets. As a result, their actions turn out to be half-hearted and not truly innovative. Then they wonder why things don't get better.

What such folks don't seem to realize is that taking the same approach to something over and over, even though the approach continually leads to dissatisfaction, makes no sense. So it's crucial for partners to challenge mindsets that keep them from moving forward. In order for something truly new to happen externally, something new also needs to happen internally.

We earlier discussed this internal aspect in terms of developing an affirmative and light frame of mind in order to create new possibilities, to innovate in and out of the bedroom. When a couple brings the right attitude to their relationship and to Cupid's Challenge, then other innovations for reducing pain and increasing sensuality have their best chance for success.

Oral sex, mutual masturbation, and use of sex aids may be exciting additions to your sexual repertoire if you and your partner are dealing with chronic pain. But they work best if they are part of a larger approach dedicated to building the most satisfying sexual relationship possible. A plan in which you dedicate yourselves to:

- Developing a positive, empowering attitude toward yourselves, your relationship, and your possibilities for effectively addressing Cupid's Challenge.
- Clear, caring communication about all aspects of your sex life and how to better it.
- Sincere mutual appreciation of one another that is consistently demonstrated both in and out of the bedroom.
- A sensual approach to sex that sees it as a delicious game to play together as opposed to some "serious" matter that you have to "get right."

Dedicating yourselves to such principles may be the most profoundly practical action that you and your partner can take in addressing Cupid's Challenge.

# Chapter Twelve

# The Arrow of Intimacy

Sex, by its nature, is a physically intimate activity. However, where the body goes, the mind and heart may not follow. Even if a couple has been together for years, they may experience only a meager emotional bond during sex. They may touch each other, have intercourse, and even find physical pleasure in doing so. Yet, both partners may feel they are in bed with a stranger.

These scenarios can be described as having two kinds of intimacy—physical and emotional—and they don't always go together. Countless partnerships, including many facing Cupid's Challenge, have the first kind of intimacy but are lacking in the second. As a result, the relationship may be deficient in sexual pleasure too. That's because the most satisfying sex is not just physically, but also emotionally intimate in which the partners feel joined in their bodies, their hearts, their heads, and their souls.

## Why Emotional Intimacy Is So Important to Good Sex

With emotional intimacy present, a couple can savor additional delights that enhance and intensify their physical pleasure. But by emotionally bonding, the partners' entire beings become involved to make for a deeper, more all-inclusive union. In particular:

- Emotional intimacy creates a positive atmosphere in which partners feel more secure, confident, and hopeful, all of which are pleasurable experiences in themselves.

- In sexual situations, feelings of closeness tend to have physiological effects that increase partners' responsiveness to each other. Their blood flows more freely to erogenous areas, their bodies become more sensitive to each other's touch, and their lubricating fluids become more copious.
- Partners find themselves caring not only about their own pleasure but also their mates. In fact, much of their enjoyment may come from knowing they are pleasing their lover. The net effect is their pleasure is doubled.
- When couples feel close, the sexual encounter serves as a confirmation of, and as a kind of exclamation point for, the relationship. It assures each partner of the other's love and binds the two even more tightly. However by failing to touch each other's deep emotions, their sex may become shallow, even boring and tedious.

In short, when partners feel emotionally close to one another, they become more than a man and a woman in a sexual union. They become lovers. For couples facing Cupid's Challenge, there are even more reasons for cultivating this emotional intimacy:

- The pleasure of feeling emotionally close can help counteract physical discomfort by releasing endorphins that make the experience of pain less wearing. (Nerve Gating)
- When partners have a close emotional bond, relatively unstressful contact such as cuddling and gentle touching may result in much physical pleasure.
- Emotional intimacy can help strengthen partners' resolve to address Cupid's Challenge in the most effective ways. Without that connection, the will to work together for the sake of each other and the relationship may be seriously weakened.
- Emotional intimacy is an essential ingredient to great sex. So, if scintillating sex is the couple's objective in addressing Cupid's Challenge, then enjoying a high level of emotional intimacy needs to be a natural part of that objective.

For all of these reasons, it's important for couples who are facing Cupid's Challenge to understand whether their degree of emotional intimacy is high, low, or somewhere in between. How do they feel about one another in bed? Is sex for them just a physical matter, or do they also derive deep emotional benefits from being sexually close? Does one of the partners want greater emotional closeness than what the other is offering?

---

Cupid's Point

Does emotional intimacy play a large part in your sexual activities? Does its presence, or absence, make a considerable difference in how much pleasure you get from sex with your partner?

Think of at least two ways in which greater emotional intimacy could help you and your partner deal more effectively with Cupid's Challenge. For example, would it enhance your communication about sex and sensuality? What other positive effects might it have?

---

If you find that you and your partner are not as emotionally close as you would like, then it's time for the two of you to consider sharpening one of Cupid's most essential approaches—the Arrow of Intimacy.

Because of its relations to other topics we've discussed, intimacy is a fine way to bring together some of the main points in the previous chapters and to learn how all of Cupid's arrows fit together into a single potent bundle as you and your partner embark on the adventure of addressing Cupid's Challenge. In particular, we can start with understanding what factors tend to create intimacy.

## The Seven Foundations of Intimacy

Emotional intimacy rests on seven foundations.

Love. This is the most fundamental basis for intimacy. For partners to feel emotionally close to one another, it's crucial that they genuinely care for each other and express their feelings through their words and actions. Each time partners express their love through what they sincerely say or do for one another, they bind themselves more closely together.

Unconditional acceptance and approval. Acceptance and approval are usually implied by love, but not always. Two people may love each other, yet not accept each other as they are. Instead, one or both may try to change their mate into their idea of what the other should be. Unconditional acceptance and approval means liking and loving your partner as he or she is. That doesn't mean you have to approve of every last thing your partner does. However, the more the two of you accept, respect, and appreciate each other's character, personality, and body, the more you tend to gravitate toward one another.

Strong mutual support. This too is usually encompassed by love, but it's so important that it's worth highlighting on its own. When life places sizable difficulties on our shoulders, it's heartening and relationship-affirming to know that our partner is ready to share the load so that we don't have to bear the burden alone. By strongly supporting each other, especially through hard times, partners build intimacy and the knowledge that they are "in this together" for better or worse.

Acceptance of differences and mutual respect. Emotional intimacy involves the wonderful mystery of how two people can become seemingly one while remaining separate individuals. It's important for partners not to expect each other to become clones of one another. In the first place, that's impossible. In the second, even if they were able to do so, they would lose their separate identities—which is what drew the individuals together in the first place. By accepting individual differences and showing respect for those differences and each other, partners affirm one another and help create a strong bond.

Communication. One of the main roadblocks to intimacy is a lack of communication. Without communication, partners can't know what the other believes, feels, desires, and hopes for. As a result, they can't understand who the other person truly is. And how can they feel genuinely close if they don't even know each other? Communication is an indispensable part of being able to create and maintain a close connection.

Sharing Life. To grow close, partners must find similar interests and spend quality time together pursuing them. By sharing enjoyable experiences and working on projects together, they make memories and create a history for themselves.

This doesn't mean they have to constantly be in each other's back pocket. Each partner will certainly have interests not shared by the other. However, they must have some substantial mutual interests and activities if they are to feel they are sharing life together.

Sexual togetherness. When partners enjoy the same sexual activities and feel comfortable with each other in bed, their physical intimacy increases. This in turn helps to create emotional intimacy. When sexual togetherness is weak, both physical and emotional closeness suffer.

---

Cupid's Point

On a sheet of paper, list the seven foundations of emotional intimacy. Beside each entry, write a score from one to ten that represents how strongly that particular foundation is reflected in your relationship. Now write a score from one to ten reflecting the degree of emotional intimacy you feel is in your relationship. Does that score agree with the average of the ones you wrote down for the seven foundations?

Which of the seven foundations contributes the most to emotional intimacy in your partnership? Which would you work on first to increase your emotional intimacy? This could be an especially revealing exercise for both you and your partner to work on and then to compare notes on.

---

These seven foundations of intimacy are important for all couples, including those facing Cupid's Challenge. If your relationship is deficient in any of these, your emotional intimacy level would benefit from strengthening them as a path to bringing you and your mate closer.

This raises an obvious question: How can you strengthen the seven foundations? What steps can you and your partner take to build a firmer base for emotional intimacy?

One excellent way is to put into practice what we've discussed earlier about Cupid's arrows. That's because each arrow we've discussed—Health, Attitude, Light, Communication, Appreciation, Touch, Romance, Innovation, and Intimacy—is closely related to one or more of the seven foundations of intimacy. As a result, when you sharpen Cupid's other arrows and make them part of your quiver, you automatically hone the Arrow of Intimacy too.

This can become clearer by looking carefully at how each of the other arrows also generate intimacy. This will help you see that the various arrows are not just a diverse group of unrelated approaches. But rather, they reinforce each other, working synergistically to build closeness so that lovers can create their strongest possible response to Cupid's Challenge.

## How Cupid's Arrows Create Emotional Intimacy

### Health Inspires Intimacy

You learned earlier that the Arrow of Health is about the chronic pain survivor becoming the primary manager of her or his pain while taking charge of their health through diet, exercise, medications, and other pertinent health-related treatments. As a result, a healthy lifestyle enhances emotional intimacy in a number of ways:

- By caring for their health, partners build self-respect. This is important because the more a person respects herself or himself, the better they are able to shift attention away from their own needs and focus more on their partner's in order to enhance intimacy.

- When couples are in better health, they feel better. They are able to approach problems together with a more positive, can-do outlook, which in turn helps generate closeness.
- Improved health also leads to more energy and stamina. This extra energy is then available for sex and other activities that unite partners. This means more opportunities for partners to share life together, which is one of the foundations of emotional intimacy.
- Better health is a pain management asset that can directly lead to more comfort and pleasure in bed.

For all of these reasons, when you and your partner develop the Arrow of Health, you are at the same time sharpening the Arrow of Intimacy.

## A Positive Attitude Inspires Intimacy

Earlier we also discussed how the Arrow of Attitude is about assuming a positive disposition toward several key aspects of Cupid's Challenge. First, it involves having an empowered attitude toward managing pain. Doing so tends to increase self-respect, which in turn strengthens our ability to express love to our partner.

Second, attitude is about partners developing a positive view of their sexual relations. By affirming themselves sexually, they build sexual togetherness. Closeness also tends to increase when partners work together to develop a model of sexual activity that pleases both.

Third, the Arrow of Attitude is concerned with partners taking a positive attitude toward themselves individually and their whole relationship. In both cases, they again build self-respect and provide each other with approval and support which brings them even closer.

## Lightness Inspires Intimacy

The Arrow of Light is about creating a light, relaxed atmosphere in the bedroom. This helps build intimacy by fostering a space where lovers can express themselves freely and enjoy one another without worry or blame.

As we discussed before, many relationships become heavy due to alienation, negative attitudes, self-ultimatums, or other reasons. And typically this heaviness results in a loss of intimacy between the partners. Remember Karl and Melissa who were having trouble returning to their former happy sex life? By putting too much pressure on themselves, they created an oppressive atmosphere in their bedroom. Instead of finding physical and emotional intimacy, they found themselves butting heads. Emotional intimacy simply doesn't do well with long faces.

However, when partners lighten up they make room for play and sensual delight. This increases sexual togetherness, a foundation for emotional intimacy. It also strengthens several other foundations, including communication, sharing life together, unconditional acceptance, and, of course, love.

Lightness can also be invaluable to intimacy outside the bedroom. For most relationships, there are enough disappointments and sorrows in the course of living without adding additional weight by taking on a heavy, gloomy disposition. Heaviness often leads to sadness, feelings of being trapped, and alienation. But by lightening up, looking at the funny side of things, and relaxing our minds when troubles encroach, we create breathing room for ourselves, our partner, and the relationship as a whole. This helps provide the psychological and emotional support on which partners can draw closer and more effectively face whatever concerns they have.

### Communication Inspires Intimacy

Communication is absolutely necessary for intimacy. It's so important that it might even be considered a foundation that helps to support all of the other foundations. The opposite is also true—intimacy inspires communication. It can do this by creating new possibilities for partners to express themselves. For example, when lovers feel close to one another, they may sense that they are in a kind of communion. No words at all may be needed. Just the touch of a hand or a look may speak volumes.

## Appreciation Inspires Intimacy

When partners express their mutual appreciation, they show their approval, respect, and love for each other. To sincerely appreciate someone through words or actions is a way of reaching out and touching that person. We tend to naturally gravitate toward those who show us sincere approval and regard, so it's no wonder that mutual appreciation tends to bring partners closer together. A few sincere and well-placed compliments or words of gratitude are truly invigorating to emotional intimacy.

## Sensual Savvy Inspires Intimacy

We also found earlier that you can increase your sensual savvy with the Arrows of Touch, Romance, and Innovation. The most obvious reason for deploying these arrows is to heighten sensuality and create more options for you and your lover to address Cupid's Challenge. However, they can also provide a powerful boost to emotional intimacy.

This may be most obvious for the Arrow of Touch because cuddling, hand-holding, and other nonsexual ways of touching help partners assure one another of their love and affection and also serve as an additional avenue for drawing them closer together. Sexual touch too can enhance emotional intimacy. By being aware of how to best sensually please each other, partners show their appreciation, respect, and love, all of which go hand in hand with intimacy.

The Arrow of Romance builds intimacy in two ways. First, it enhances sexual togetherness. By creating a bedroom atmosphere that pleases all of the senses, partners can intensify their sexual experience, which tends to draw them closer emotionally. Second, romance is about sharing life together, which is one of the seven foundations of intimacy. When couples kindle their romance by sharing special times, they get more in tune with one another and walk more closely together down the road of life.

Finally, the Arrow of Innovation helps build intimacy by increasing partners' sexual togetherness. When lovers explore the positions and activities that can provide them the most pleasure, even when experiencing chronic pain, they are focusing on how to optimize their sexual compatibility. Greater intimacy also comes about from the partners working together, providing each other with mutual support as they address a shared problem.

## Interlocking Arrows and Dimensions

The linkage between the Arrows of Health, Attitude, Light, Communication, Appreciation, Touch, Romance, Innovation, and Intimacy is far-reaching. For example:

Attitude Affects Health. A positive, empowering attitude can be one of a couple's most important assets as they work toward achieving their very best health. Some ways in which attitude influences health include:

- Greater energy levels.
- More ability to fight disease.
- Added willingness to see a physician.
- Stronger commitment to following a health improvement program.

Appreciation Affects Communication. When partners feel appreciated by one another, they are more willing to communicate about issues that affect them singularly and as a couple. If one or both of them feel underappreciated, then anger, disappointment, and other negative emotions may distort attempts to communicate.

Lightness Affects Innovation. Cultivating a light, sensual atmosphere in the bedroom helps partners explore new possibilities openly and with a hopeful frame of mind. Conversely, a heavy atmosphere can make exploration feel like work instead of pleasure.

Communication Affects Just About Everything! The Arrow of Communication is closely related to *all* of Cupid's other arrows. For example, creating a light atmosphere and expressing appreciation both require good communication between partners. Clear, caring communication is such a major part of sharpening every arrow that it may be your most important asset as you face Cupid's Challenge. As long as you and your lover commit yourselves to clear, caring communication, and keep a strong positive attitude, you have an excellent opportunity to achieve the satisfying sex life you desire.

---

### Cupid's Point

What other ways are Cupid's Arrows interrelated? For example, how might the Arrow of Touch strengthen the Arrow of Appreciation? And since the Arrow of Romance includes enjoying special times together, how could that affect the Arrow of Attitude or the Arrow of Innovation?

---

Maybe you've noticed that this special interlocking nature of Cupid's arrows is particularly good news for couples coping with Cupid's Challenge. It's good news because it means that all of the arrows reinforce one another. So, by sharpening one arrow, you also sharpen other arrows. As a result, any time you make an improvement to one aspect of Cupid's Challenge, you simultaneously make progress with others too.

On the other side of the coin, the interlocking nature of Cupid's arrows also implies that if any arrow happens to be dull in your relationship, it may negatively affect other aspects of your lives together. For example, less romance detracts from attitude, touch, and other aspects of your partnership just as less communication negatively affects all aspects.

These close connections among the arrows also relate to the four dimensions—the physical, psychological, relational, and sensual—of chronic pain challenges in couples' sex lives as illustrated below:

- The Arrow of Health → the physical dimension.
- The Arrows of Attitude and Light → the psychological dimension.

- The Arrows of Communication and Appreciation → the relational dimension.
- The Arrows of Touch, Romance, Innovation, and Intimacy → the sensual dimension.

Now we're in a position to see that because of the interlocking and reinforcing nature of the arrows, each one actually influences all four dimensions in one way or another. Appreciation, for example, is important not only for the relationship as a whole but also for the physical and sensual dimensions. Romance doesn't affect only sensuality. It also has an impact on the relational and psychological dimensions.

All of this serves to bring us back full circle to one of the main themes discussed throughout this book—Cupid's Challenge is a *multidimensional* challenge. So, your best strategy is to deal with it multidimensionally, which means giving every one of Cupid's arrows its proper due. In that way, you and your partner will be better able to formulate your most powerful response to the disruption chronic pain is causing to your sex life.

Conclusion

Cupid's wonderful arrows can be summarized in a few simple but all-important principles. These can serve you and your partner well if you commit yourselves to practicing them every single day and night as you two move forward into the more sensually pleasing, intimate, and satisfying sex life that you desire and deserve. Here are Cupid's arrows in a nutshell:

- Above all, take care of your health.
- Cultivate an empowering attitude.
- Take a light, sensual approach to sex and Cupid's Challenge.
- Appreciate each other and show your appreciation abundantly.
- Build your sensual savviness and closeness through touch, romance, innovation, and intimacy.
- Communicate, communicate, communicate.

# Appendix A

# Making A Better Choice: Dietary Guidelines

Every day we face important health choices. Among the most vital of these are the choices we make for our diet. Too often, we choose what to eat and drink based solely on what sounds tasty to us at the time or what is most convenient to prepare or purchase, and pay little attention to what our body signals would be preferable for us to eat.

Unfortunately, there is a widespread belief that what's good for us at the table will be bland and unsatisfying. But that's simply not true. There are increasingly many dietary choices that are simple, delicious, and healthy. To make those choices may require stopping for a moment and thinking about what we are doing, but that small effort can be rewarded many times over through better health, increased energy, and greater longevity.

The following are some basic guidelines and suggestions to help you get started in making better dietary choices. With the increasing awareness about the link between the food we eat and our wellbeing, I encourage you to seek out even more information about reducing your sugar intake, adding more plant-based foods to your meals, and managing your weight, among other related topics.

**BREAKFAST.** Start your day with a healthy, protein-rich breakfast, a solid meal that can increase your metabolism while providing you with plenty of energy for the day ahead. Say no to:

- Grapefruit and a piece of toast, or nothing at all (too light).
- Sugar donuts, pancakes and syrup, or a three-egg cheese omelet
- Hash browns (too heavy and too sweet).
- Cold or hot cereals.

Say yes to any of the following:
- Two boiled eggs.
- Two scrambled eggs with one ounce of cheese.
- One egg, one slice of cheese, and salsa all rolled into a corn tortilla.
- Two slices of Canadian bacon with cheese rolled into a corn tortilla.
- Two scrambled, yolkless eggs.
- Two patties of lean sausage.
- A protein shake, or add a small glass of fruit juice or a cup of decaffeinated coffee sweetened with Stevia.

**LUNCH.** A healthy lunch helps keep you alert and energetic throughout the afternoon. Again, don't make your meal too light or too heavy. Choose a lunch that is high in protein and not weighed down in fats, sugars, or too many carbohydrates. Make sure it has enough caloric content to provide you with afternoon energy. Say no to:
- A single six-ounce low-fat yogurt cup (too light).
- A typical fast food restaurant double cheeseburger with fries and a sugary soft drink (too heavy).

Say yes to any of the following:
- One or two roll-ups consisting of lean turkey with a slice of white cheese, Dijon mustard, and lettuce; add an apple for dessert.
- A four-ounce lean hamburger patty with a tomato and half a cup of corn tortilla chips.

- A salad consisting of four ounces of lean ham, an ounce of white cheese, one or two boiled egg whites, lettuce, tomato, cucumber, and one to two tablespoons of light dressing.

In general, try to have four ounces of protein with your lunch, which may be in the form of fish, chicken, red meat, or veal. Include a salad, a cooked vegetable, or both. If you want to have a carbohydrate, this is the best time of the day to have one cup of pasta, rice (preferably brown), or potatoes. For a drink, consider water, Crystal Light, or decaffeinated tea.

**MID-AFTERNOON SNACK.** If needed, an afternoon pick-me-up can consist of a snack with substantial protein content, a piece of fresh fruit, or fresh vegetables. Make your snack low in saturated fats and processed sugars. Say no to:

- Candy bars, donuts, sugared soft drinks, French fries, corn chips, and potato chips.

Say yes to any of the following:

- One six-ounce cup of low-fat yogurt.
- Fresh fruit, such as a medium apple or a cup of mixed fruit.
- One quarter cup of nuts—cashews are generally lowest in fat, pecans highest, and almonds and walnuts in the middle.
- A high-protein drink or bar.

*Remember to drink fluids throughout the day.* These can be in the form of water, or for flavor try Mio or exogenous ketones from www.mcmnutrition.com, or flavored, preferably decaffeinated, iced teas with a noncaloric sweetener. For active days when you may be out working in your yard or playing golf, be sure not to get dehydrated. To replenish minerals and electrolytes, Add an ampule of fulvic and humic from www.drinkdurt.com/meridian to improve your electrolyte balance and enhance your absorption of minerals and vitamins.

**DINNER.** Dinner is best as the lightest meal of the day. This is because the after-dinner segment of the day is generally when we are least active. Dinner is advised to include at least one vegetable or a salad, or both, and about four ounces of protein. Say no to:

- An eight-ounce steak, steak fries, and a piece of apple pie.
- Simple carbohydrate dishes such as potatoes, bread, pastas, or rice.

Say yes to:

- A four-ounce cut of lean beef steak, salmon, or chicken along with one cup of a green vegetable and/or a garden salad dressed lightly.

*Still hungry after any of your meals?* If so, have a glass of water and wait for a half hour. That's about how long it takes for the tummy to catch up with the brain and register satisfaction.

These suggestions are meant to give you a feel for the kinds of meals and proportion choices that can have a positive impact on your health. Don't feel tied to the specific menu items mentioned. Make equivalent substitutions to fit your own tastes.

While the general portions suggested will approximate the needs of many individuals, they are not written in stone. Optimum daily caloric intake depends on your height, body structure, age, activity level, and base metabolism. Work with your physician or dietician to determine what's right for you and adjust portions to your specific needs. The idea is not necessarily to go on a weight-loss diet, but to change your eating lifestyle to optimize your health and longevity.

Underlying these choices are some general principles that are worthwhile repeating:

- Choose complex over simple carbohydrates.
  Avoid processed sugars; for sweetening, choose a noncaloric sweetener.
  Enjoy fresh fruits and vegetables.

Prefer whole grains over processed grains.

- Minimize saturated fats.

  Choose lean cuts of meat.

  Choose foods and oils high in unsaturated fats. These include nuts, and oils such as canola and olive.

  Check the labels of processed foods for their fat content and choose foods low in saturated fat.

- Make sure you are getting enough high quality protein.

  Vary your diet with different kinds of meat and fish.

  Choose lean over fatty cuts of meat.

  Fish is an excellent source of protein, but limit your intake to no more than two helpings a week. Check with your doctor about what's optimal for you.

- Limit your intake of salt.

  Get in the habit of reading labels to determine the sodium content of the foods you purchase.

  Find tasty non-salt substitutes to spice up your foods. These days, there are more and more tasty sodium-free and low-sodium seasonings available.

- Limit your caffeine consumption.

  Decaffeinated coffees and teas are now widely available.

  Instead of iced tea, consider substituting with a drink that has no or minimal caffeine, such as water or some other non-sugary beverage.

REMEMBER: What you eat is one of the main determinants of your wellbeing. Many people find they lose ten or more pounds in a fairly short time following the simple suggestions above. Consistently making wise dietary choices can go a very long way toward helping you look, feel, and live your best.

# Appendix B

# Choosing A Doctor

Building a positive, trusting, and forward-looking relationship with your healthcare provider is a crucial aspect of your total wellbeing. To develop such a relationship, your important initial step is to choose your doctor or dentist wisely.

## Overall Qualities to Seek

- *Your health care provider must be Qualified, Competent, Caring, and Committed to your health.*
- *He or she must be concerned about your patient history.* When you visit a new doctor or dentist, you bring with you a history of experiences with other healthcare professionals. This history may be less than fully positive. It may include inadequate results, increased pain, feelings of self-consciousness, or the sense that you were not listened to or even believed. Your new health care provider needs to be interested in your specific concerns about past experiences as well as your current health concerns.
- *He or she must be dedicated to providing you with positive, predictable results.* Your new doctor or dentist needs to be eager to work with you to build mutual trust and respect in part by providing sufficient time to understand your specific health situation. If you are dealing with health problems, he or she needs to provide a detailed treatment plan. This will include careful goal setting, reassurance, and an emphasis on the responsibilities of both patient and doctor for enacting the plan.

## Criteria to Remember in Searching for a Health Care Provider

1. When searching for a new doctor or dentist, pay close attention to referrals:

- Referrals may come from family, friends, co-workers, or neighbors. They may also come from other doctors or medical associations.
- Pay special attention to referrals from current or former patients. The highest compliment for a health care professional is a referral from a satisfied patient.
- But remember, *you* are the final judge of the suitability of a doctor or dentist for you.

2. When you first call a physician's office, does office staff:
- Seem genuinely caring over the phone?
- Treat you with friendliness and respect?
- Ask you questions about how they can best serve your needs?
- Provide you with the information that you request?

3. When you first visit a new doctor or dentist: Are you offered the opportunity for a telemedicine or in-person visit?
- In an in-person visit are you given an office tour during which you are introduced to office staff?
- If you ask for testimonials, are you satisfied with the reply? (Remember that patients must give a physician permission to use their name and story.)
- Physicians today will have websites on which they provide information about themselves, their office, and their vision. This can be a good source of information about the doctor, and may include testimonials. Consider taking a look at their FaceBook or Instagram account if public, do they look like and act like someone you would want to share with

- Does the doctor keep the appointment time? If he or she is running behind a few minutes, are you promptly notified? Do office staff members courteously provide you with a healthy snack or beverage when you have to wait as a way to show that they understand the value of your time and patience?
- Does the doctor listen to you attentively? Is he or she genuinely interested in your specific condition and in your overall health?
- Does the doctor take an interest in you as a person?
- Is the doctor dedicated to providing a complete, effective, treatment strategy or plan for your optimal health?

4. Even after you have chosen a doctor, it's important to keep asking questions:
- In later visits, does the doctor continue to listen carefully to you and communicate clearly?
- Does he or she continue to provide effective goal setting with a positive treatment plan?
- Do you like and trust this doctor? Do you feel comfortable that you are in good hands? Do you like the results you are getting?
- How about the office staff? Do they continue to show courtesy, friendliness, and professionalism at every visit?
- Does the office staff follow up with you after every procedure? Does the doctor call you personally after a procedure or a change in medications?
- Does the doctor and the staff quickly reply to your phone messages and emails?

Overall, your experience with the doctor and the office should consistently confirm that you have made the right choice. As you move forward, remember that the best doctor-patient relationships are built on mutual respect and clear communication coming from both sides of the desk.

# We Care About You

For free information on how you can learn to thrive, follow us for the most up to date information @everydayhealthhacker and @meridianhealthinstitute. Subscribe to our podcast Everyday Health Hacker™ on your favorite platform or YouTube Dr. Liza Leal. We would love to hear from you and appreciate your comments and questions.